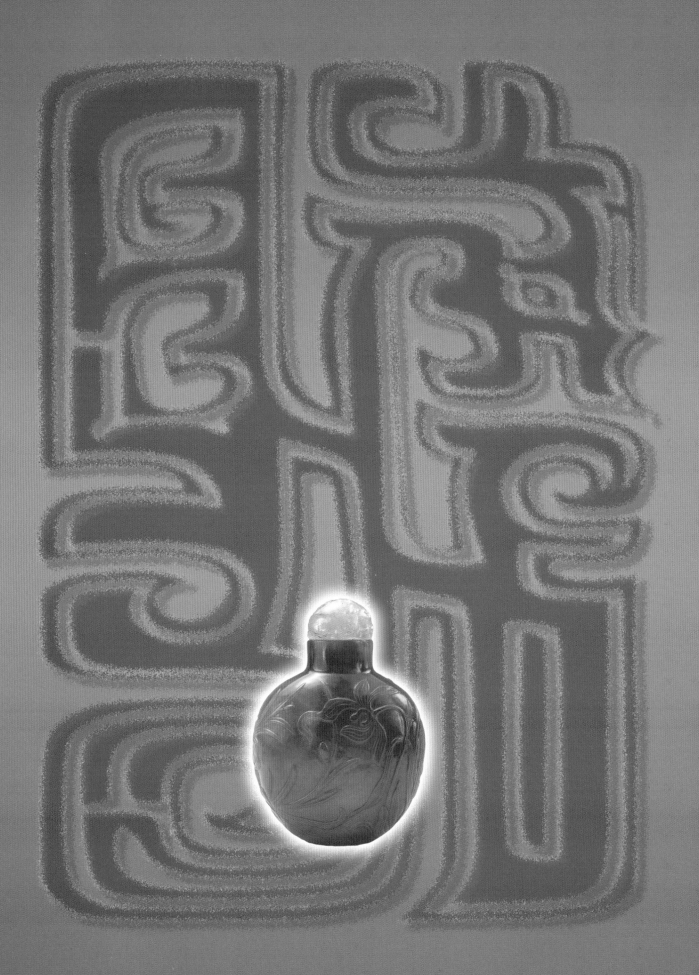

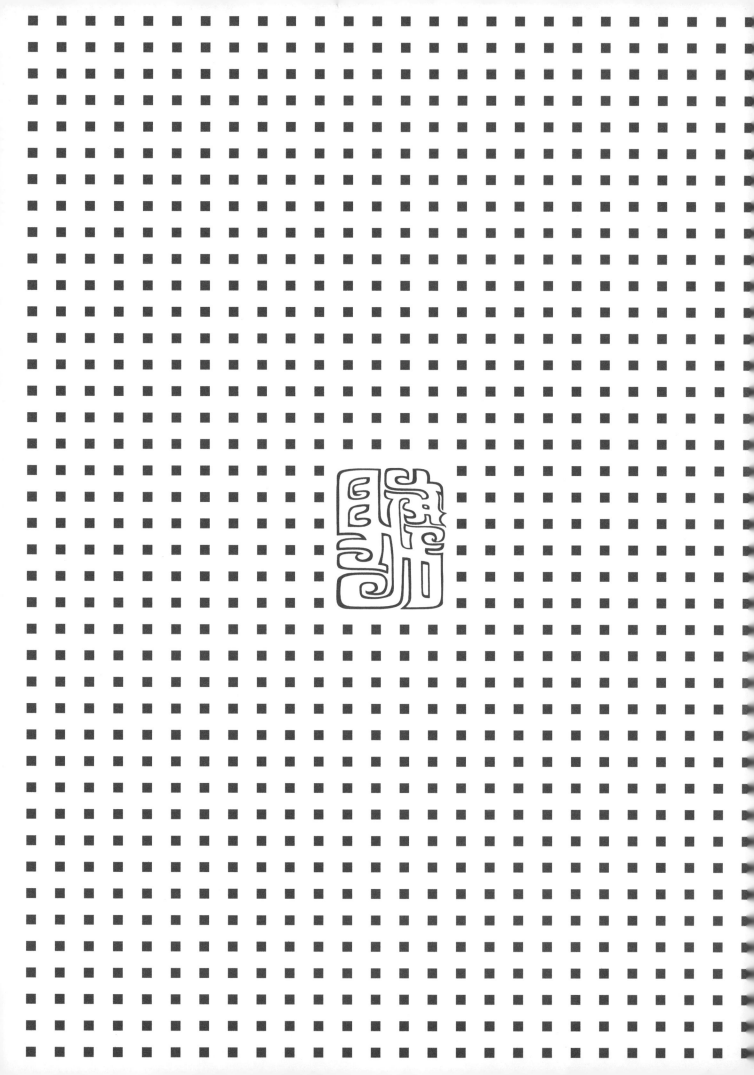

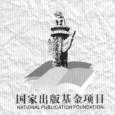
国家出版基金项目
NATIONAL PUBLICATION FOUNDATION

中华医药卫生

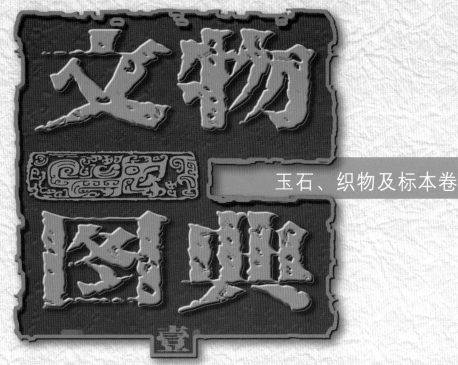

文物图典

玉石、织物及标本卷

壹

主　编　李经纬　梁　峻　刘学春
总主译　白永权
主　译　范晓晖　陈　曦

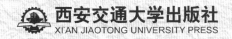
西安交通大学出版社
XI'AN JIAOTONG UNIVERSITY PRESS

图书在版编目 (CIP) 数据

中华医药卫生文物图典 . 1. 玉石、织物及标本卷 . / 李经纬，

梁峻，刘学春主编 . — 西安：西安交通大学出版社，2016.12

ISBN 978-7-5605-7016-7

Ⅰ . ①中… Ⅱ . ①李… ②梁… ③刘… Ⅲ . ①中国医药学—

玉石—中国—图录②中国医药学 – 编织物 – 中国 – 图录③中国

医药学 – 标本 – 中国 – 图录 Ⅳ . ① R–092 ② K870.2

中国版本图书馆 CIP 数据核字（2015）第 022436 号

书　　名	中华医药卫生文物图典（一）玉石、织物及标本卷
主　　编	李经纬　梁　峻　刘学春
责任编辑	张沛烨

出版发行　西安交通大学出版社

　　　　　（西安市兴庆南路 10 号　邮政编码 710049）

网　　址　http://www.xjtupress.com

电　　话　（029）82668805 82668502（医学分社）

　　　　　（029）82668315（总编办）

传　　真　（029）82668280

印　　刷　中煤地西安地图制印有限公司

开　　本　889mm×1194mm　1/16　印张 32.75　字数　531 千字

版次印次　2017 年 12 月第 1 版　2017 年 12 月第 1 次印刷

书　　号　ISBN 978-7-5605-7016-7

定　　价　980.00 元

铭记感受历史

自信自重自强

书贺

中华医药卫生文物图典问世

陈可冀 谨题

二〇一七年肖

陈可冀　中国科学院院士、国医大师

精修醫藥衛生文物

圖典功著當代

深究岐黄學術思想

淵源惠澤千秋

中華醫藥衛生文物圖典出版志慶

丁酉孟秋 孫光榮 敬題於北京

孙光荣　国医大师

中華醫藥 衛生文物圖典出版

彰顯中醫藥
文化精神

体现中医药
歷史价值

歲次丁酉夏 王琦

王琦　国医大师

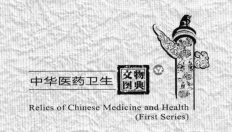

中华医药卫生文物图典（一）
丛书编撰委员会

主　编　李经纬　梁　峻　刘学春

副主编　廖　果　吴鸿洲　康兴军　和中浚　刘小斌　杨金生

　　　　　郑怀林　徐江雁　白建疆　黄　煌

编　委　李洪晓　梁永宣　王强虎　董树平　马　健　王　霞

　　　　　张雅宗　朱德明　包哈申　张建青　郑　蓉　庄乾竹

　　　　　李宏红　刘哲峰　王宏才　陈润东

总主译　白永权

主　译　陈向京　聂文信　范晓晖　温　睿　赵永生　杜彦龙

　　　　　吉　乐　李小棉　郭　梦　陈　曦

副主译（按姓氏音序排列）

　　　　　董艳云　姜雨孜　李建西　刘　慧　马　健　任宝磊

　　　　　任　萌　任　莹　王　颇　习通源　谢皖吉　徐素云

　　　　　许崇钰　许　梅　詹菊红　赵　菲　邹郝晶

译　者（按姓氏音序排列）

迟征宇　邓　甜　付一豪　高　琛　高　媛　郭　宁

韩　蕾　何宗昌　胡勇强　黄　鋆　蒋新蕾　康晓薇

李静波　刘雅恬　刘妍萌　鲁显生　马　月　牛笑语

唐云鹏　唐臻娜　田　多　铁红玲　佟健一　王　晨

王　丹　王　栋　王　丽　王　媛　王慧敏　王梦杰

王仙先　吴耀均　席　慧　肖国强　许子洋　闫红贤

杨姣姣　姚　晔　张　阳　张　鋆　张继飞　张梦原

张晓谦　赵　欣　赵亚力　郑　青　郑艳华　朱江嵩

朱瑛培

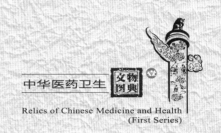

Relics of Chinese Medicine and Health
(First Series)

本册编撰委员会

主　编　李经纬　梁　峻　刘学春

副主编　廖　果　吴鸿洲　康兴军　和中浚　刘小斌　杨金生

　　　　　郑怀林　徐江雁　白建疆　黄　煌

编　委　李洪晓　梁永宣　王强虎　董树平　马　健　王　霞

　　　　　张雅宗　朱德明　包哈申　张建青　郑　蓉　庄乾竹

　　　　　李宏红　刘哲峰　王宏才　陈润东

总主译　白永权

主　译　范晓晖　陈　曦

副主译　任　莹　王　颇

译　者　田　多　王仙先　付一豪　赵　菲　马　月

丛书策划委员会

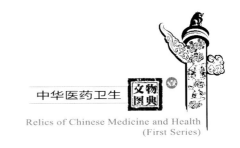

中华医药卫生 文物图典

Relics of Chinese Medicine and Health
(First Series)

序 言

　　探索天、地、人运动变化规律以及"气化物生"过程的相互关系，是人类永恒的课题。宇宙不可逆，地球不可逆，人生不可逆业已成为共识。天地造化形成自然，人类活动构成文化。文物既是文化的载体，又是物化的历史，还是文明的见证。

　　追求健康长寿是人类共同的夙愿。中华民族之所以繁衍昌盛，健康文化起了巨大的推动作用。由于古人谋求生存发展、应对环境变化产生的智慧，大多反映在以医药卫生为核心的健康文化之中，所以，习总书记说："中医药学是中国古代科学的瑰宝，也是打开中华文明宝库的钥匙"。

　　秉持文化大发展、大繁荣理念，中国中医科学院李经纬、梁峻等为负责人的科研团队在完成科技部"国家重点医药卫生文物收集调研和保护"课题获 2005 年度中华中医药学会科技二等奖基础上，又资鉴"夏商周断代工程""中华文明探源工程"等相关考古成果，用有重要价值的新出土文物置换原拍摄质量较差的文物，适当补充民族医药文物，共精选收载 5000 余件。经西安交通大学出版社申报，《中华医药卫生文物图典（一）》（以下简称《图典》）于 2013 年获得了国家出版基金的资助，并经专业翻译团队翻译，使《图典》得以面世。

　　文物承载的信息多元丰富，发掘解读其中蕴藏的智慧并非易事。医药卫生文物更具有特殊性，除文物的一般属性外，还承载着传统医学发展史迹与促进健康的信息。运用历史唯物主义观察发掘文物信息，善于从生活文物中领悟卫生信息，才能准确解读其功能，也才能诠释其在民生健康中的历史作用，收到以古鉴今之效果。"历史是现实的根源"，任何一个民族都不能割断历史，史料都包含在文化中。"文化是民族的血脉，是人民的精神家园"，文化繁荣才能实现中华民族的伟大复兴。值本《图典》付梓之际，用"梳理文化之脉，必获健康之果"作为序言并和作者、读者共勉！

中央文史研究馆馆员
中国工程院院士　王永炎
丁酉年仲夏

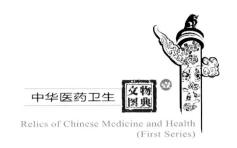

中华医药卫生 文物图典

Relics of Chinese Medicine and Health
(First Series)

前 言

　　文化是相对自然的概念，是考古界常用词汇。文物是文化的重要组成部分，既是文明的物证，又是物化的历史。狭义医药卫生文物是疾病防治模式语境下的解读，而广义医药卫生文物则是躯体、心态、环境适应三维健康模式下的诠释。中华民族是56个民族组成的多元一体大家庭，中华医药卫生文物当然包括各民族的健康文化遗存。

　　天地造化如造山、板块漂移、气候变迁、生物起源进化等形成自然。气化物生莫贵于人，即整个生物进化的最高成果是人类自身。广义而言，人类生存思维留下的痕迹即物质财富和精神财富总和构成文化，其一般的物化形式是视觉感知的文物、文献、胜迹等。其中质变标志明晰的文化如文字、文物、城市、礼仪等可称作文明。从唯物史观视角观察，狭义文化即精神财富，尤其体现人类精、气、神状态的事项，其本质也具有特殊物质属性，如量子也具有波粒二相性，这种粒子也是物质，无非运动方式特殊而已。现代所谓可重复验证的"科学"，事实上也是从文化中分离出来的事项，因此也是一种特殊文化形式。追求健康长寿是人类共同的夙愿。中华民族之所以繁衍昌盛，是因为健康文化异彩纷呈。中华优秀传统医药文化之所以博大精深，是因为其原创思维博大、格物致知精深，所以，习总书记说："中医药学是中国古代科学的瑰宝，也是打开中华文明宝库的钥匙"。

文化既反映时代、地域、民族分布、生产资料来源、技术水平等信息，又反映人类认知水平和生存智慧。发掘解读文物、文献中蕴藏的健康知识和灵动智慧，首先是从事健康工作者的责任和义务。《易经》设有"观"卦，人类作为观察者，不仅要积极收藏展陈文物，而且要善于捕捉文物倾诉的信息，汲取养分，启迪思维，收到古为今用之效果。墨子三表法，首先一表即"本之于古者圣王之事"，也是强调古代史实的重要性。"历史是现实的根源"，现实是未来的基础。任何一个国家、地区、民族都不能割断历史、忽略基础，这个基础就是文化。"文化是民族的血脉，是人民的精神家园"。文化繁荣才能驱动各项事业发展，才能实现中华民族的伟大复兴。

人类从类人猿分化出来。"禄丰古猿禄丰种"是云南禄丰发现的类人猿化石，距今七八百万年。距今200万年前人类进入旧石器时代，直立行走，打制石器产生工具意识，管理火种，是所谓"燧人氏"时代。中国留存有更新世早、中期的元谋、蓝田、北京人等遗址。距今10万—5万年前，人类进入旧石器时代中期，即早期智人阶段，脑容量增加，和欧洲、非洲人种相比，原始蒙古人种颧骨前突等，是所谓"伏羲氏"时代。中国发现的马坝、长阳、丁村人等较典型。距今5万—1万年前，人类进入旧石器时代晚期，即晚期智人阶段，细石器、骨角器等遍布全国，山顶洞、柳江、资阳人等较典型。

中石器时代距今约1万年，是旧石器时代向新石器时代的短暂过渡期，弓箭发明，狗被驯化。河南灵井、陕西沙苑遗址等作为代表。距今1万—公元前2600年前后，人类进入新石器时代，磨光石器、烧制陶器，出现农业村落并饲养家畜，是所谓"神农氏"时代。公元前7000年以来，在甲、骨、陶、石等载体上出现契刻符号、七音阶骨笛乐器等，反映出人文气息趋浓。公元前6000—公元前3500年的老官台、裴李岗、河姆渡、马家浜、仰韶等文化遗址，彰显出先民围绕生存健康问题所做的各种努力。

公元前4800年以来，以关中、晋南、豫西为中心形成的仰韶文化，是中原史前文化的重要标志。以半坡、庙底沟类型为典型，自公元前3500年走向繁荣，属于锄耕粟黍稻兼营渔猎饲养猪鸡经济方式，彩陶尤其发达。公元前4400—公元前3300年，长江中游的大溪文化，薄胎彩陶和白陶发达。公元前4300—公元前2500年山东丰岛的大汶口文化，红陶为主。公元前3500年前后，辽东的红山文化原始宗教发展。公元前 3300 年以来，长江下游由河姆渡、马家浜文化衍续的良渚文化和陇西的马家窑文化、江淮间的薛家岗文化时趋发达。

公元前 2600—公元前 2000 年，黄河中下游龙山文化群形成，冶铸铜器，制作玉器，土坯、石灰、夯筑技术开始应用。公元前 2697 年，轩辕战败炎帝（有说其后裔）、蚩尤而为黄帝纪元元年。黄帝西巡访贤，"至岐见岐伯，引载而归，访于治道"。其引归地"溱洧襟带于前，梅泰环拱于后"，即今河南新密市古城寨。岐黄答问，构建《黄帝内经》健康知识体系，中华文明从关注民生健康起步。颛顼改革宗教，神职人员出现；帝喾修身节用，帝尧和合百国，舜同律度量衡，大禹疏导治水，中华民族不断繁衍昌盛。

公元前 2070 年，禹之子启以豫西晋南为中心建立夏王朝，二里头青铜文化为其特征，半地穴、窑洞、地面建筑并存。饮食卫生器具、酒器增多。朱砂安神作用在宫殿应用。公元前 1600 年，商灭夏。偃师商城设有铸铜作坊。公元前 1300 年，盘庚迁殷，使用甲骨文。武丁时期青铜浑铸、分铸并存。公元前 1056 年，相传周"文王被殷纣拘于羑里，演《周易》，成六十四卦"。公元前 1046 年，武王克商建周，定都镐京。青铜器始铸长篇铭文，周原发掘出微型甲骨文字。公元前 770 年，平王东迁。虢国铸铜柄铁剑。公元前 753 年，秦国设置史官。公元前 707 年出现蝗灾、公元前 613 年出现"哈雷彗星"，均被孔子载入《春秋》。公元前 221 年，秦始皇统一中国，多元一体民族大家庭形成，中华医药卫生文物异彩纷呈。

中国是治史大国，历来重视发展文化博物事业，1955 年成立卫生部中医研究院时就设置医史研究室，1982 年中国医史文献研究所成立时复建中国医史博物馆研究收藏展陈文物。2000—2003 年，经王永炎院士、姚乃礼院长等呼吁，科技部批准立项，由李经纬、梁峻为负责人的团队完成"国家重点医药卫生文物收集调研和保护"项目任务，受到科技部项目验收组专家的高度评价，获中华中医药学会科技进步二等奖。2013 年，在国家出版基金资助下，课题组对部分文物重新拍摄或必要置换、充实民族医药文物后，由西安交通大学出版社编辑、组聘国内一流翻译团队英译说明文字付梓，受到国家中医药博物馆筹备工作领导小组和办公室的高度重视。

"物以类聚"，《图典》主要依据文物质地、种类分为 9 卷，计有陶瓷，金属，纸质，竹木，玉石、织品及标本，壁画石刻及遗址，少数民族文物，其他，备考等卷。同卷下主要根据历史年代或小类分册设章。每卷下的历史时段不求统一。遵循上述规则将《图典》划分为21册，总计收载文物5000余件。对每件文物的描述，除质地、规格、馆藏等基本要素外，重点描述其在民生健康中的作用。对少数暂不明确的事项在括号中注明待考。对引自各博物馆的材料除在文物后列出馆藏外，还在书后再次统一列出馆名或参考书目，以充分尊重其馆藏权，也同时维护本典作者的引用权。

21世纪，围绕人类健康的生命科学将飞速发展，但科学离不开文化，文化离不开文物。发掘文物承载的信息为现实服务，谨引用横渠先生四言之两语："为天地立心，为生民立命"，既作为编撰本《图典》之宗旨，也是我们践行国家"一带一路"倡议的具体努力。希冀通过本《图典》的出版发行，教育国人，提振中华民族精神；走向世界，为人类健康事业贡献力量。

李经纬　梁峻　刘学春

2017年6月于北京

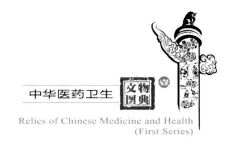

中华医药卫生 文物图典

Relics of Chinese Medicine and Health
(First Series)

目 录

第二章 织 品

第三章　标　本

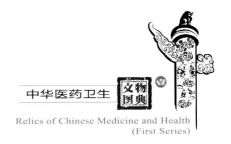

中华医药卫生
Relics of Chinese Medicine and Health
(First Series)

Contents

Chapter Two   Textiles

Chapter Three   Specimens

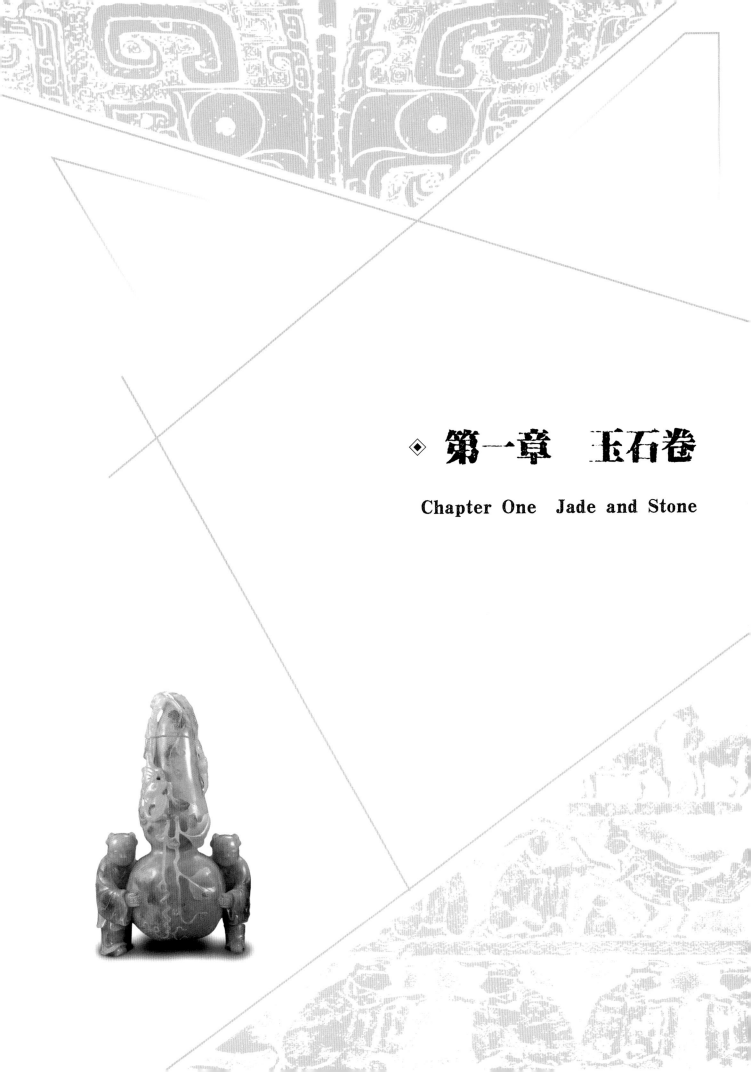

第一章　玉石卷

Chapter One　Jade and Stone

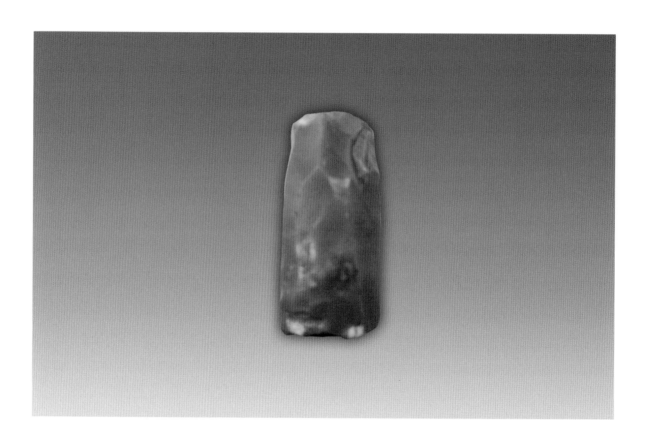

玉阳具

旧石器时代

石质

长 2.9 厘米，直径 1.5 厘米

Stone Male Genitalia

The Paleolithic Age

Stone

Length 2.9 cm/ Diameter 1.5 cm

石祖为细腻石材通体雕琢而成的男性生殖器形状，是生殖崇拜时期的祭祀用品。先民们相信祭祀供奉石祖有助于传宗接代、维系族类不断发展壮大的作用，后被中医祝由科所传承。

张雅宗藏

The artifact, made of fine whole rock material, is shaped like a male genitalia, or phallus, which was a sacrificial item during the period of reproduction worship. The ancestors believed that consecrating the phallus during sacrificial ceremony helped reproduction and constant growth of their clans. The tradition was later inherited by the department of incantation and psychology in Traditional Chinese Medicine.

Collected by Zhang Yazong

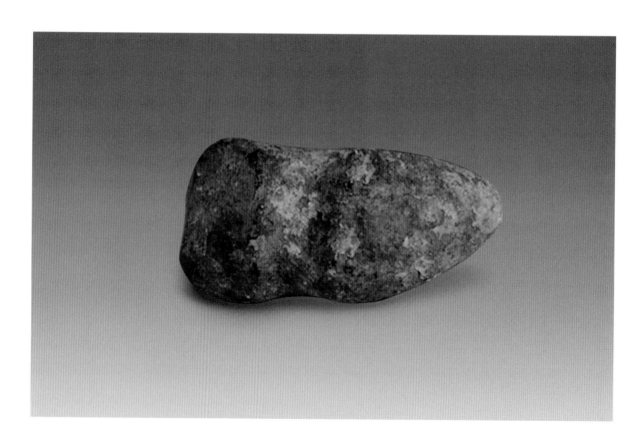

石祖

新石器时代

石质

长 16 厘米，直径 7 厘米，重 1500 克

Stone Phallus

The Neolithic Age

Stone

Length 16 cm/ Diameter 7 cm/ Weight 1,500 g

呈男性生殖器状。为图腾崇拜器物。陕西省
洛南县征集。

陕西医史博物馆藏

The phallus is shaped like a male genitalia for
totemism. It was collected in Luonan County,
Shaanxi Province.

Preserved in Shaanxi Museum of Medical History

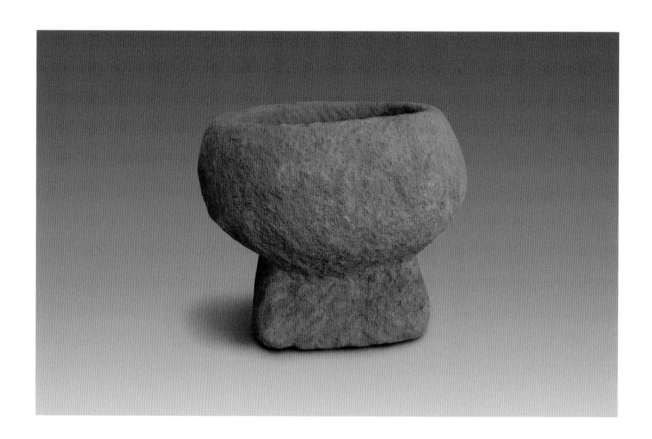

石臼

新石器时代

石质

口径 20 厘米，底径 16 厘米，通高 20 厘米，重 11200 克

Stone Mortar

The Neolithic Age

Stone

Mouth Diameter 20 cm/ Bottom Diameter 16 cm/ Height 20 cm/ Weight 11,200 g

敛口，鼓腹，圜底，下有方形足。制药工具。

陕西省澄城县征集。

陕西医史博物馆藏

The stone mortar has a contracted mouth, a bulged belly, a round base, and a square foot. It was utilized for preparing medicine. The mortar was collected in Chengcheng County, Shaanxi Province.

Preserved in Shaanxi Museum of Medical History

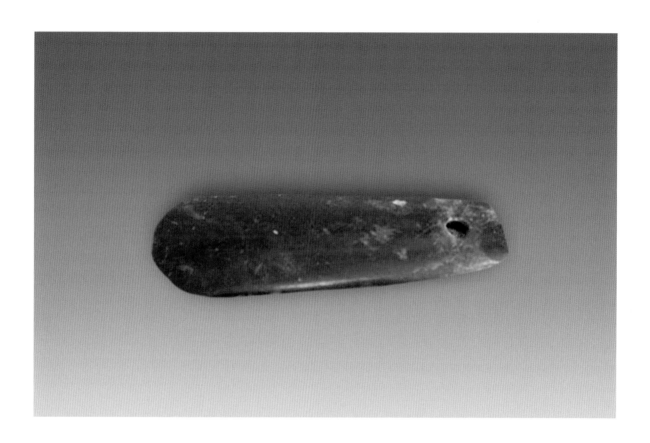

玉锛

新石器时代

石质

长 20.5 厘米，宽 9.5 厘米，重 400 克

Jade Adze

The Neolithic Age

Stone

Length 20.5 cm/ Width 9.5 cm/ Weight 400 g

铲状，一头处有一圆孔。1/3 处有断裂痕。

生产工具。陕西省西安市灞桥征集。

陕西医史博物馆藏

The adze is shaped like a spade with a round hole at one end. It was used as a labor tool and breaks appear at one third of the length. It was collected from Baqiao District of Xi'an, Shaanxi Province.

Preserved in Shaanxi Museum of Medical History

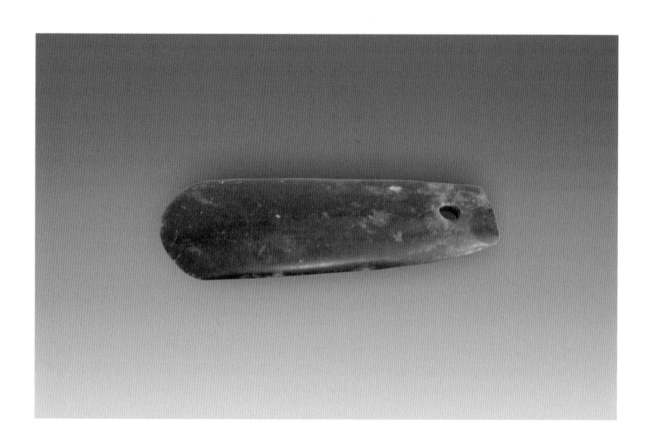

玉锛

新石器时代

石质

长 15 厘米，宽 4 厘米，重 160 克

Jade Adze

The Neolithic Age

Stone

Length 15 cm/ Width 4 cm/ Weight 160 g

铲状，一端有 1.5 厘米的圆孔。生产工具。

完整无损。陕西省咸阳市秦都区征集。

陕西医史博物馆藏

The adze is shaped like a spade with a round
hole of 1.5 cm in diameter at one end. It was
used as a labor tool. It is still in good condition.
It was collected from Qindu District of Xi'an,
Shaanxi Province.

Preserved in Shaanxi of Museum Medical History

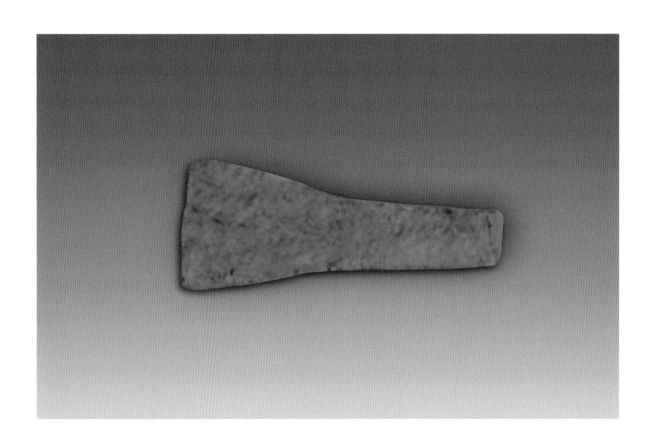

石锛

新石器时代

石质

长 7.5 厘米，宽 2 厘米，高 1 厘米，重 100 克

Stone Adze

The Neolithic Age

Stone

Length 7.5 cm/ Width 2 cm/ Height 1 cm/ Weight 100 g

呈楔形状。生产工具。有残。

陕西医史博物馆藏

The stone adze is wedge-shaped and incomplete.

It was used as a labor tool.

Preserved in Shaanxi of Museum Medical History

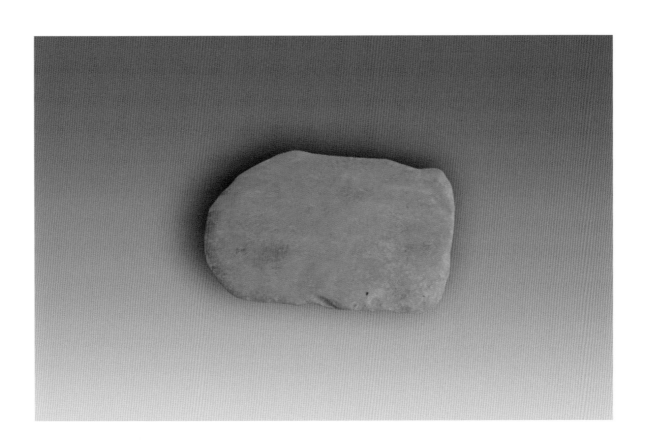

石锛

新石器时代

石质

长 20.1 厘米，宽 10.7 厘米，重 1300 克

Stone Adze

The Neolithic Age

Stone

Length 20.1 cm/ Width10.7 cm/ Weight 1,300 g

铲状。生产工具。完整无损。陕西省澄城县
征集。

陕西医史博物馆藏

The stone adze is shaped like a spade. It was used
as a labor tool and is still in good condition. It was
collected from Chengcheng County, Shaanxi
Province.

Preserved in Shaanxi Museum of Medical History

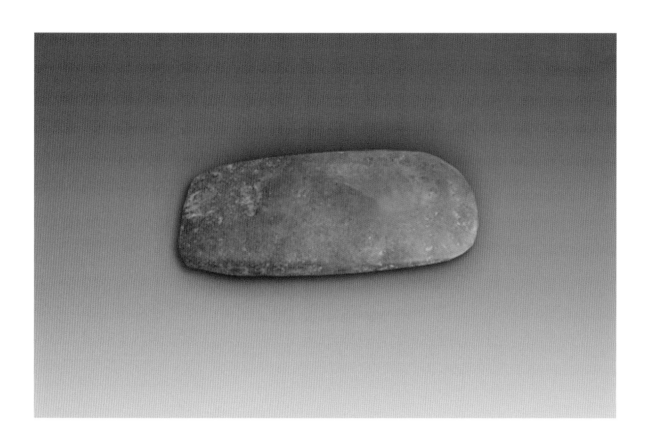

石锛

新石器时代

石质

长 27 厘米，宽 13 厘米，厚 3.5 厘米，重 3600 克

Stone Adze

The Neolithic Period

Stone

Length 27 cm/ Width 13 cm/ Thickness 3.5 cm/ Weight 3,600 g

扁状，一头较锋利。生产、生活器具。完整无损。

陕西医史博物馆藏

The stone adze is flat with a sharp edge at one end. It has been used as a labor tool or a living utensil. It is still in good condition.

Preserved in Shaanxi Museum of Medical History

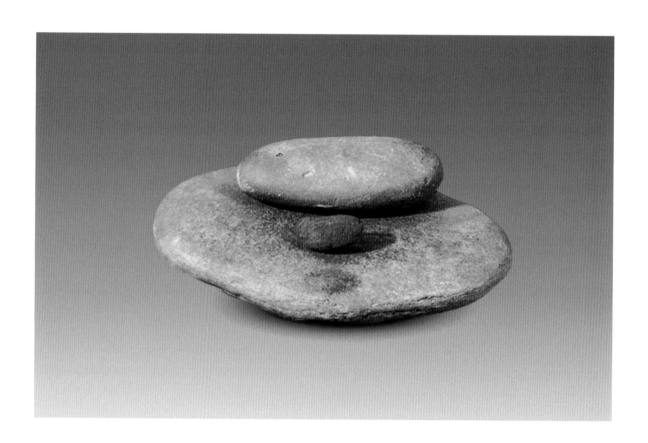

石质研磨盘

新石器时代

石质

磨盘：长 15 厘米，宽 11 厘米

Stone Grinding Pan

The Neolithic Age

Stone

Grinding Pan: Length 15 cm/ Width 11 cm

由磨盘和磨棒组成，磨盘呈扁平状，中部略凹陷；磨棒呈近圆柱状。二者表面均较光滑，有明显研磨痕迹。用于研磨谷物、药物或颜料。拉萨曲贡新石器时代晚期遗址出土。

西藏博物馆藏

The collection consists of a grinding pan and a stick. The pan is flat and slightly sunken in the middle while the stick is nearly cylindrical. Both of their surfaces are smooth with clear traces of grinding. It was utilized for processing grain, medicine or pigments. This artifact was excavated at the Late Neolithic Age site in Qugong, Lhasa.

Preserved in Tibet Museum

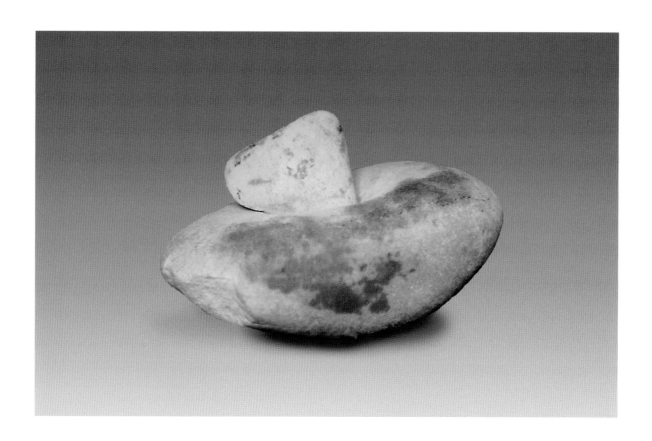

药臼

新石器时代

石质

臼：长 27 厘米，高 11 厘米

Medicine Mortar

The Neolithic Age

Stone

Molar: Length 27 cm/ Height 11 cm

石臼由天然卵石稍经加工制成，呈不规则扁圆形，中部凿磨出凹陷。带石杵一件，也为自然石块。用以捣碎药物。西安市十里铺新石器遗址出土。

陕西医史博物馆藏

This mortar is made of natural pebble by moderate processing. It is irregularly oblate with a concave in the middle part. The stone pestle, which is also made of natural stone, was used for mushing medicine. The collection was excavated at a site of the Neolithic Age in Shilipu, Xi'an City, Shaanxi Province.

Preserved in Shaanxi Museum of Medical History

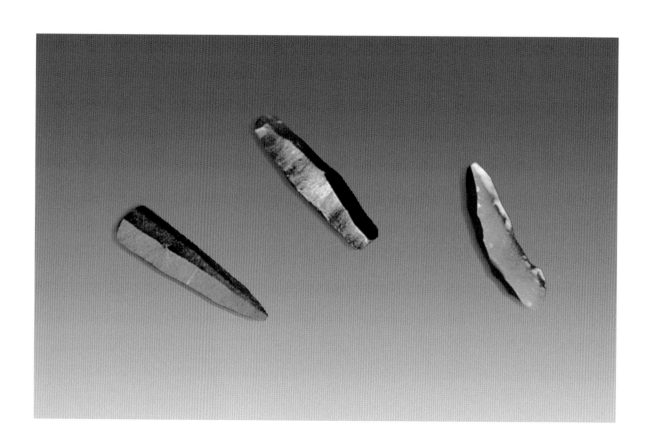

玛瑙石叶

新石器时代

石质

长约 2 厘米

Stone Leaves

The Neolithic Age

Stone

Length about 2 cm

该藏品包括细石叶 3 件，均为柳叶状，其中
1 件为绿色，2 件为褐色，均为细腻坚硬的
石质剥片而成，两侧有刃。可用于放血、破痈。

陕西医史博物馆藏

The collection consists of three fine stone
leaves, which are all shaped like a willow leaf:
a green one and two ochre ones. All are made
of fine and hard rock stripping, with blade on
both sides. They were used for bloodletting and
breaking carbuncles.

Preserved in Shaanxi Museum of Medical History

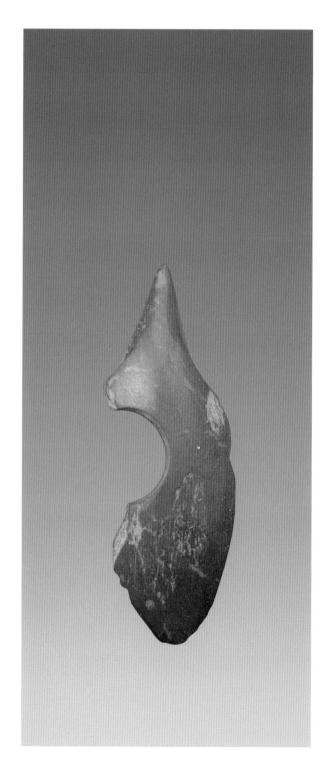

泗水石古砭

新石器时代

石质

长 8.2 厘米，宽 2.7 厘米

Ancient Stone Needle Made of Sishui Stone

The Neolithic Age

Stone

Length 8.2 cm/ Width 2.7 cm

石砭系用细腻石材通体磨制而成，平面近叶形，一端长而尖，中部有圆形穿孔，穿孔一侧边缘残缺。可能是医用器具石砭。

张雅宗藏

The stone needle, ground out of fine whole rock material, has a leaf-shaped plane with one long and sharp end. In the middle there is a round hole with broken rim on one side. The artifact might be a stone needle for medical purposes.
Collected by Zhang Yazong

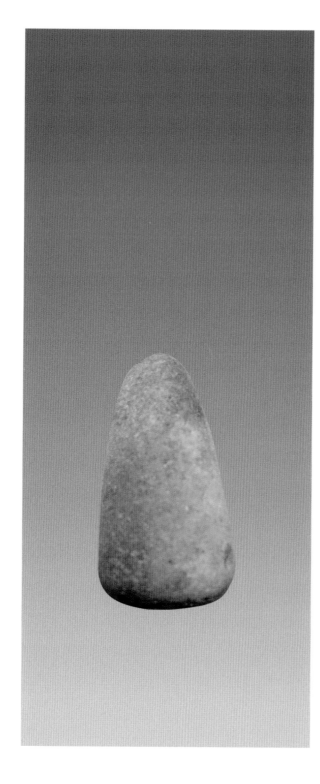

熨石砭

新石器时代

石质

长 5.3 厘米，宽 2.7 厘米

Heating Stone Needle

The Neolithic Age

Stone

Length 5.3 cm/ Width 2.7 cm

近圆锥体形，用砂岩通体磨制而成，器形规整。可能是新石器时代远古先民用于穴位治疗以及热敷患处的原始工具，是在"砭"未形成之前的原始雏形。

张雅宗藏

The nearly cone-shaped needle with regular form was ground out of a whole sandstone. It might be a primary tool used by primitive people in the Neolithic Age for acupoint treatment and hot compressing of the affected area. It was a primitive rudiment of stone needle.

Collected by Zhang Yazong

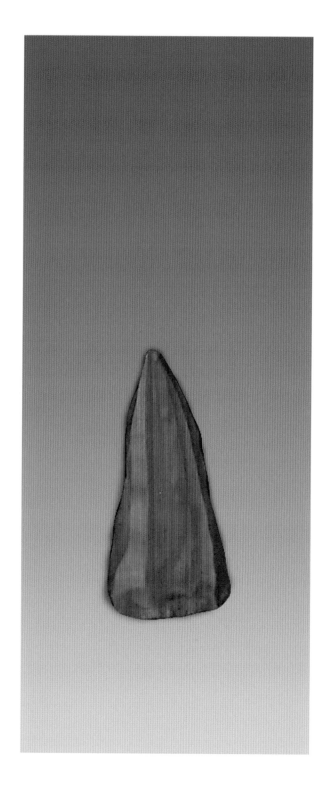

砭石

新石器时代

石质

长 3.6 厘米，宽 1.8 厘米，厚 0.6 厘米

Stone Needle

The Neolithic Age

Stone

Length 3.6 cm/ Width 1.8 cm/ Thickness 0.6 cm

暗灰色硅质岩打制成的锥状石核。表面光滑，
有明显的使用痕迹。医用。

　　中华医学会 / 上海中医药大学医史博物馆藏

The needle is made of the coniform corestone of
dark gray siliceous rock. The surface is smooth
with clear traces of using. It was used for medical
purposes.

Preserved in Chinese Medical Association/ Museum
of Chinese Medicine, Shanghai University of
Traditional Chinese Medicine

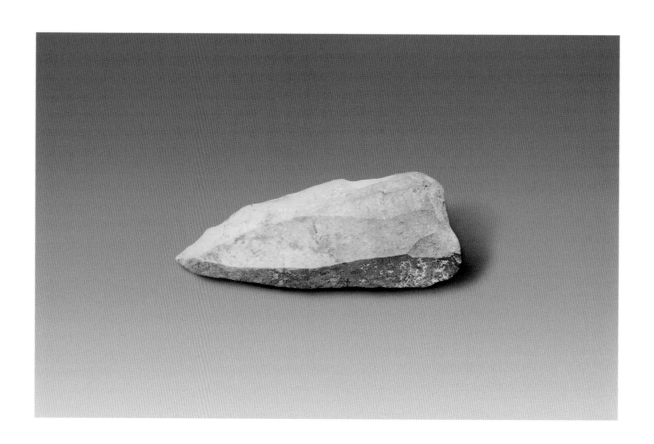

砭石

新石器时代

石质

长 7 厘米，宽 3 厘米

Stone Needle

The Neolithic Age

Stone

Length 7 cm/ Width 3 cm

石片打制成的尖状器，尖端锋利，两侧有刃。可用以放血、破痈、去腐肉。20 世纪 70 年代出土于河南淅川下王岗仰韶文化遗址。

陕西医史博物馆藏

The needle, which is made of stone flakes, has a sharp end, with blade on both sides. It was used for bloodletting, breaking carbuncles, and removing carrion. The needle was unearthed in Xiawanggang Yangshao Culture site in Xichuan, Henan Province, in the 1970s.

Preserved in Shaanxi Museum of Medical History

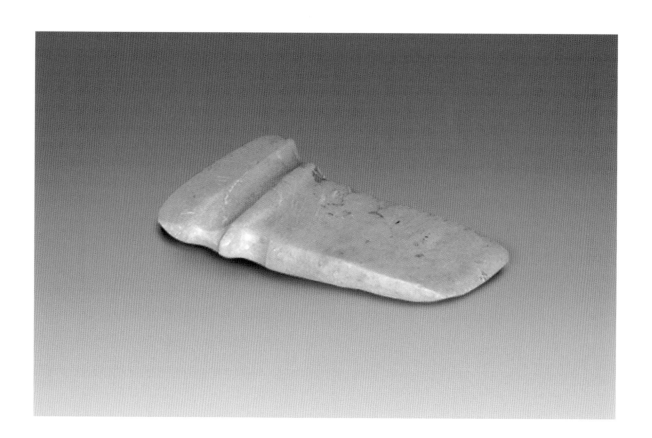

砭石

新石器时代

石质

长 8.8 厘米，宽 4 厘米，重 100 克

Stone Needle

The Neolithic Age

Stone

Length 8.8 cm/ Width 4 cm/ Weight 100 g

斧状，一边较锋利，另一端有固定用的凹槽。
白色，磨制光滑规整。为生活器具或医疗器
具。陕西省西安市蒋志坚捐赠。

陕西医史博物馆藏

The stone needle is axe-shaped with a sharp end
and a groove for fixation at the other end. It is
white and ground smoothly and structured for
medical or household daily use. The stone needle
was donated by Jiang Zhijian from Xi'an, Shaanxi
Province.

Preserved in Shaanxi Museum of Medical History

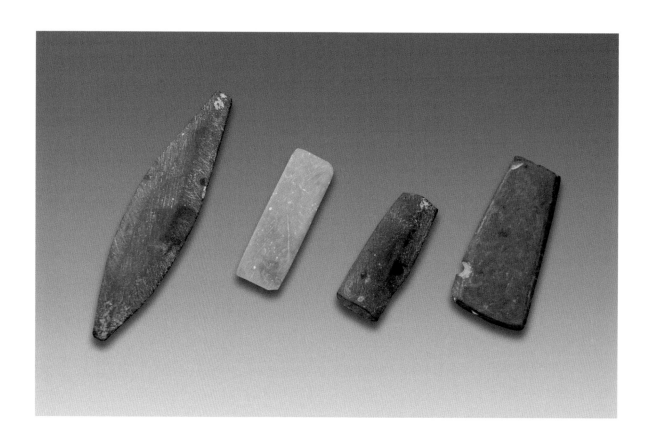

石质小刀

新石器时代

石质

长 2～4.9 厘米，宽 1.5～2.3 厘米

Stone Knives

The Neolithic Age

Stone

Length 2-4.9 cm/ Width 1.5-2.3 cm

4件，菱形、长方形或梯形，通体磨制规整、
光滑，一端有刃。属于医工混用器，以器型
判断，主要用于小型外科手术。

张雅宗藏

The four diamond-shaped, rectangular, or
trapezoid knives with a blade on one end are
regular and smooth. As a tool used in medical
profession, they were mainly used in minor
surgeries judging from their size and shape.
Collected by Zhang Yazong

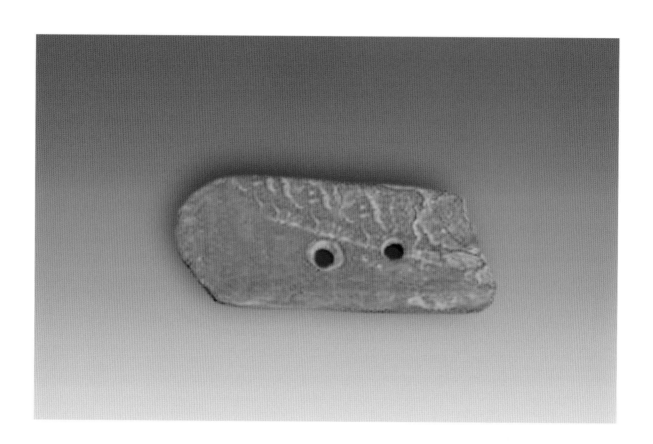

石刀

新石器时代

石质

长 10 厘米，宽 4.5 厘米，高 0.5 厘米，重 200 克

Stone Knife

The Neolithic Age

Stone

Length 10 cm/ Width 4.5 cm/ Height 0.5 cm/ Weight 200 g

匕状头，下部两边开刀。生活、生产工具。

完整无损。陕西省西安市灞桥征集。

陕西医史博物馆藏

The stone knife has a dagger-shaped head with sharp edges on both sides and is still in good condition. The stone relic was used as a labor tool or a living utensil. It was collected from Baqiao District of Xi'an in Shaanxi Province.

Preserved in Shaanxi Museum of Medical History

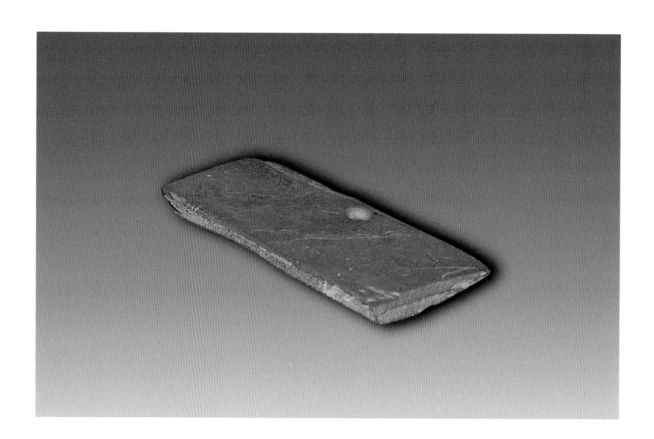

石刀

新石器时代

石质

长 10.2 厘米，宽 5 厘米，重 60 克

Stone Knife

The Neolithic Age

Stone

Length 10.2 cm/ Width 5 cm/ Weight 60 g

长方形，一边较锋利，中间有一小圆孔。生
产工具。完整无损。陕西省渭南市征集。

陕西医史博物馆藏

The stone knife is in rectangular shape. It has
only one sharp edge on which there is a small
round hole in the middle. It was used as a labor
tool. It is still in good shape. It was collected
from Weinan City, Shaanxi Province.

Preserved in Shaanxi Museum of Medical History

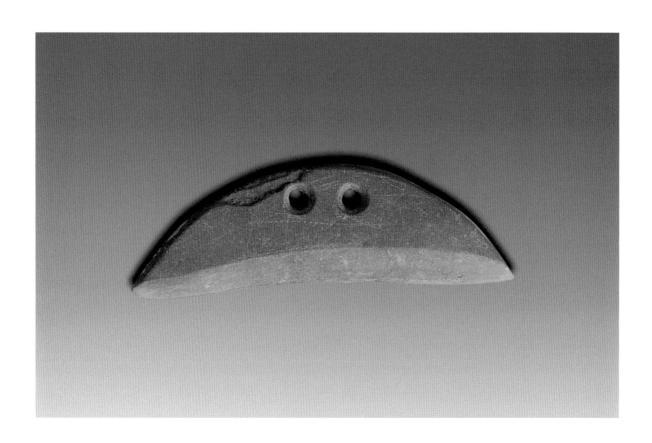

半月形石刀

新石器时代

石质

刃宽 9.5 厘米

Half-moon-shaped Stone Knife

The Neolithic Age

Stone

Blade Width 9.5 cm

青灰色页岩通体磨制而成，表面光滑。弧背，

直刃略凹，背部有 2 个钻孔。属于良渚文化。

象山县文物管理委员会藏

The stone knife is made of bluish grey shale
ground with a smooth surface. It has an arc back
with two drilled holes and a straight edge with a
slight concave. The knife belongs to the Liangzhu
Culture.

Preserved in Xiangshan County Administration
Committee of Cultural Relics

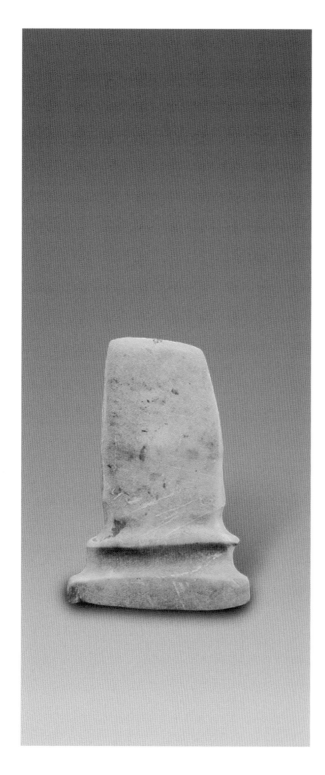

砭石

新石器时代

石质

长 10 厘米，宽 5 厘米

Stone Needle

The Neolithic Age

Stone

Length 10 cm/ Width 5 cm

斧状，一边较锋利，另一端有固定用的凹槽。

白色，磨制光滑规整。仰韶时期先民们的生

产工具，也可用于破痈、排脓。1964 年出土

于陕西省西安市浐河西岸。

陕西医史博物馆藏

The stone needle is axe-shaped with a sharp end
and a groove for fixation at the other end. It is
white and polished smoothly and structured. As an
important tool of production in Yangshao Period,
it could also be used to break carbuncles and
drain abscess. The stone needle was unearthed at
the west bank of Chan River in Xi'an, Shaanxi
Province, in 1964.

Preserved in Shaanxi Museum of Medical History

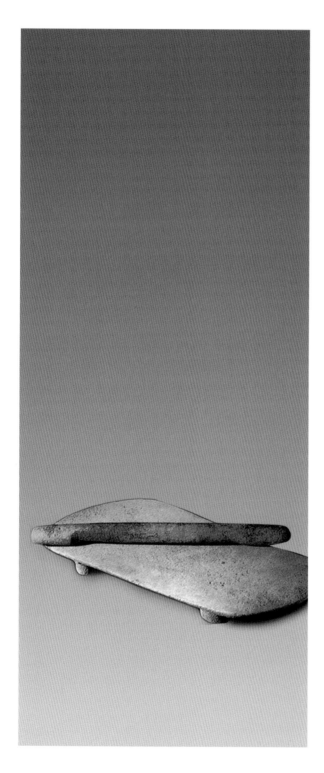

石磨盘、磨棒

新石器时代

石质

磨盘：长68厘米，宽37.5厘米，高6厘米

磨棒：长58厘米

Stone Millstone and Grinding Rod

The Neolithic Age

Stone

Millstone: Length 68 cm/ Width 37.5 cm/ Height 6 cm

Rod: Length 58 cm

磨盘由黄色砂岩通体琢磨而成，整体呈板状，平面椭圆形，前宽后窄，中部略凹陷，底部雕琢有四个柱状短足。磨棒也由砂岩磨制成圆柱形，中部较粗，两端略细。该藏是距今7000多年的裴李岗文化的典型器物，属于加工谷物等的工具。1977年河南省新郑市裴李岗出土。

河南博物院藏

The tabular millstone is made of a yellow ground sandstone. It has an elliptical surface, and wider in the front, narrower at the back, and slightly dented in the middle. It is supported by four short polished feet of cylindrical shape. The cylindrical grinding rod is also made of sandstone. It is thick in the middle and slightly thin at both ends. The collection, a typical utensil of the Peiligang Culture dated back to more than 7,000 years, was a grain-processing tool. It was unearthed at Peiligang Culture in Xinzheng City, Henan Province, in 1977.

Preserved in Henan Museum

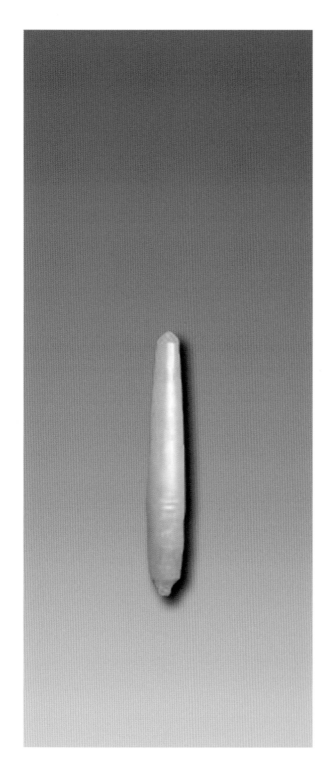

玉锥

新石器时代

玉质

长 6.1 厘米，断面边长 0.7 厘米

Jade Cone

The Neolithic Age

Jade

Length 6.1 cm/ Side Length of Cross Section 0.7 cm

翠青色玉，磨制精细。方体，下端饰浅浮雕，

圆榫带细孔，方形锥尖。1997 年浙江省海盐

县龙潭港遗址出土。

中国海盐博物馆藏

The emerald green jade cone is in the shape of
cube with a pyramidal tip. It is finely polished.
The lower part is decorated with bas-reliefs and
there is a round tenon with a tiny hole at the end.
It was excavated at Longtan Port Site of Haiyan
County, Zhejiang Province, in 1997.
Preserved in China Sea-salt Museum

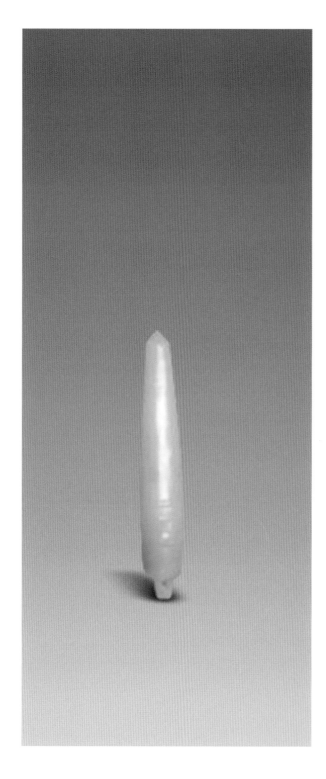

玉锥

新石器时代

玉质

长 5.7 厘米，断面边长 0.9 厘米

Jade Cone

The Neolithic Age

Jade

Length 5.7 cm/ Side Length of Cross Section 0.9 cm

翠青色玉，磨制精细。方体，下端饰浅浮雕，圆榫带细孔，方形锥尖。1997 年浙江省海盐县龙潭港遗址出土。

中国海盐博物馆藏

The emerald green jade cone is finely polished in the shape of cube with a pyramidal tip. The lower part is decorated with bas-reliefs. There is also a round tenon with a tiny hole in the lower part. It was excavated at Longtan Port Site of Haiyan County, Zhejiang Province in 1997. Preserved in China Sea-salt Museum

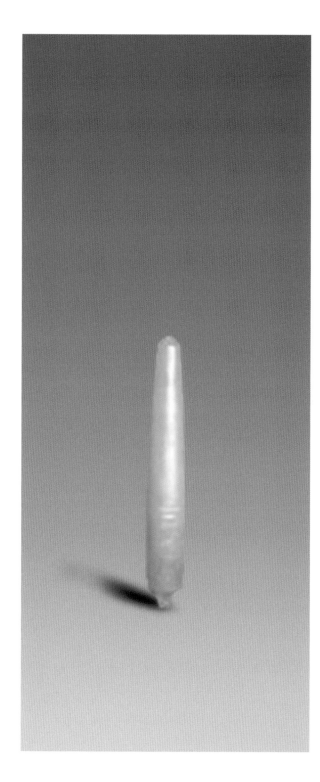

玉锥

新石器时代

玉质

长 6.1 厘米，断面边长 0.7 厘米

Jade Cone

The Neolithic Age

Jade

Length 6.1 cm/ Side Length of Cross Section 0.7 cm

翠青色玉，磨制精细。方体，下端饰浅浮雕，
圆榫带细孔，方形锥尖。1997 年浙江省海盐
县龙潭港遗址出土。

中国海盐博物馆藏

The emerald green jade cone is finely polished
in the shape of cube with a pyramidal tip. The
lower part of is decorated with bas-reliefs.
There is also a round tenon with a tiny hole in
the lower part. It was excavated at Longtan Port
Site of Haiyan County, Zhengjiang Province, in
1997.

Preserved in China Sea-salt Museum

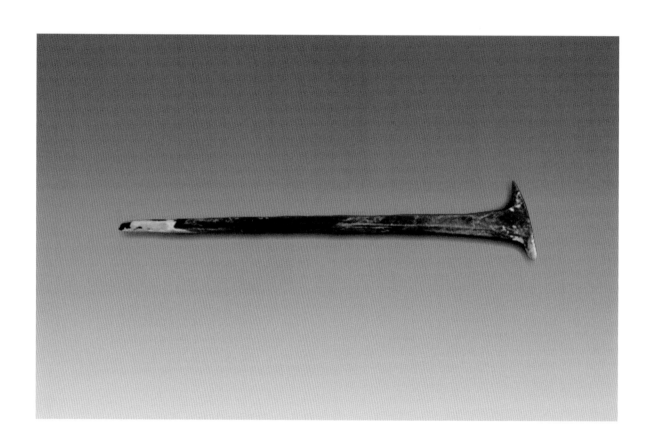

玉锥

新石器时代

玉质

长 19.5 厘米，重 29 克

Jade Cone

The Neolithic Age

Jade

Length 19.5 cm/ Weight 29 g

通体磨制而成，锥形，锥尖残，锥把头扁平。
生活器具。陕西省渭南市征集。

陕西医史博物馆藏

The entire body of the cone was ground into
cone shape, with a flat handle and a damaged
tip. The cone is an appliance for daily use, was
collected from Weinan City, Shaanxi Province.
Preserved in Shaanxi Museum of Medical History

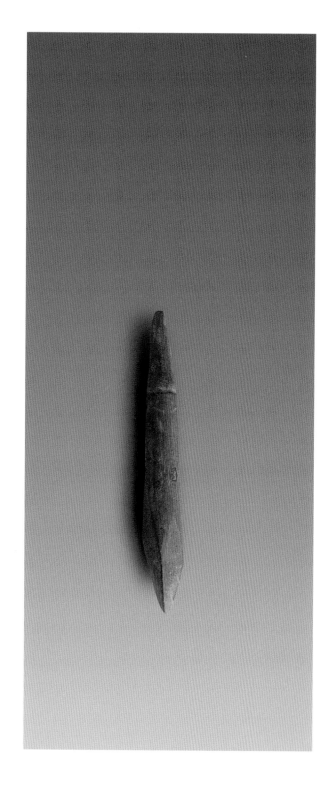

石锥

新石器时代

石质

长 6.9 厘米

Stone Cone

The Neolithic Age

Stone

Length 6.9 cm

通体磨制光滑，一端呈锥尖状，另一端有一
周弦纹，可能作系绳之用。属于河姆渡文化
第四期的遗物。可用于放血、破痈。

象山县文物管理委员会藏

The cone has a smoothly polished surface, with a
conical tip at one end and a circle of string lines at
the other which might be used as a tether. The
awl belonged to the four phases of the Hemudu
Culture and was used for bloodletting and
breaking carbuncles.

Preserved in Xiangshan County Administration
Committee of Cultural Relics

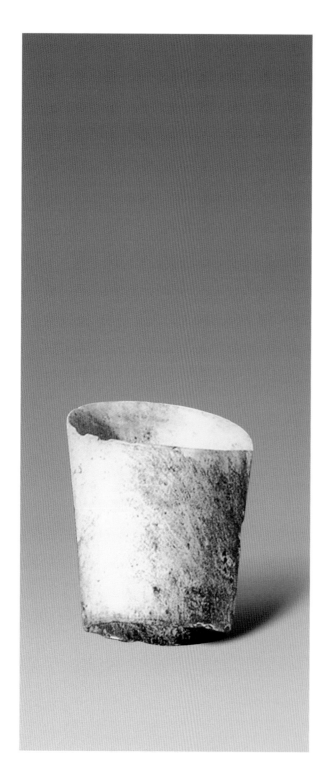

玉护臂

新石器时代

玉质

口径 5.8～7.4 厘米，高 15.5 厘米

Jade Arm Guard

The Neolithic Age

Jade

Mouth Diameter 5.8-7.4 cm/ Height 15.5 cm

护臂呈倒置的马蹄形。上端磨成斜坡形口，
且有刃。下端齐平，边沿对钻双孔，可穿系。
器壁光滑匀薄，制作精致。为技击时臂上实
用之护器。红山文化的遗物。1979 年辽宁省朝
阳市凌源县（今凌源市）出土。

辽宁省博物馆藏

The arm guard is shaped like an inverted horseshoe.
The upper end was ground into a slope-shaped
mouth with blade. Along the edge of the flat
bottom there are two drilled holes. The smooth
and thin wall shows exquisite craftmanship. The
cone was a practical arm protector in attacking
and defending. The collection is a relic of the
Hongshan Culture. It was unearthed in Lingyuan
County (now Lingyuan City), Chaoyang City,
Liaoning Province, in 1979.
Preserved in Liaoning Provincial Museum

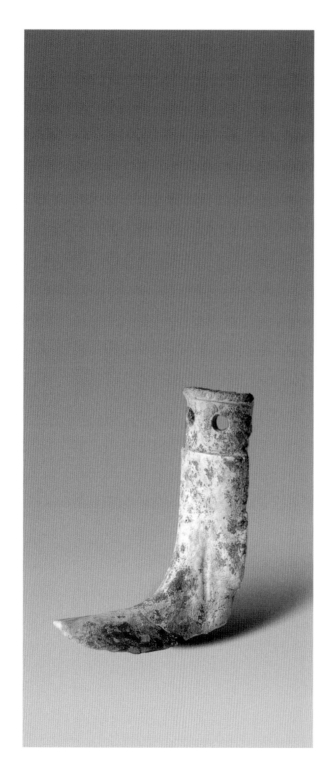

鹿角靴形器

新石器时代

角质

宽 2.9 厘米，高 7.3 厘米

Antler Boot-shaped Utensil

The Neolithic Age

Horn

Width 2.9 cm/ Height 7.3 cm

由鹿角切割磨制而成，灰褐色。侧视形态呈
靴形，一端较尖，另一端有两个穿孔。

中国海盐博物馆藏

The taupe utensil, made of ground antlers, is like a
boot when seen from the side. It is pointed at one
end and has two holes at the other end.
Preserved in China Sea-Salt Museum

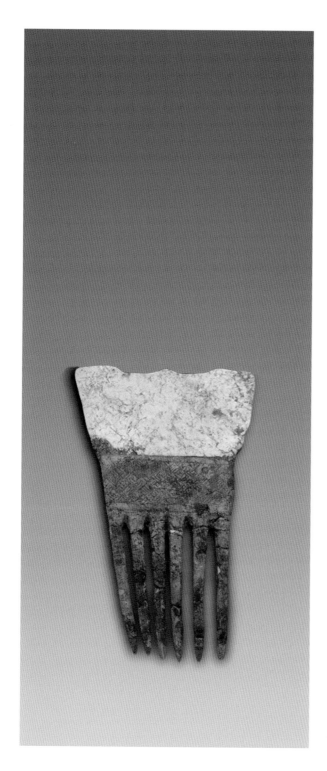

玉背象牙梳

新石器时代

玉质，象牙质

玉背：顶宽 6.4 厘米

象牙梳：顶宽 4.7 厘米，厚 0.6 厘米，通高

10.5 厘米

Ivory Comb with Jade Back

The Neolithic Age

Jade and ivory

Jade Back: Top Width 6.4 cm

Ivory Comb: Top Width 4.7 cm/ Thickness 0.6 cm/

Height 10.5 cm

整器由玉背与象牙梳镶嵌组合而成。玉背为玉冠状饰，素面，嵌于象牙梳顶端，以两枚横向销钉固定。象牙梳为六齿，顶部有阴线细刻席纹与云雷纹的组合纹饰。此器是目前良渚文化中发现的唯一一件梳子，不仅基本解决了玉冠状饰的功能问题，而且对良渚玉器研究的定位也将产生重大影响。1999 年 8 月浙江省海盐县周家浜遗址出土。

中国海盐博物馆藏

The collection consists of an ivory comb and a jade back. The jade back, crown decoration with nothing on it, is embedded by two lateral pins with the top of the ivory comb. The ivory comb has six comb teeth and has finely carved basket patterns combined with thunder cloud patterns at the top. This is the only comb in the Liangzhu Culture that has been discovered. It not only solved the problem of jade's crown-decoration function, but also has a significant impact on the orientation of Liangzhu jade research. The comb was unearthed at Zhoujiabang Site in Haiyan City, Zhejiang Province, in August 1999.

Preserved in China Sea-salt Museum

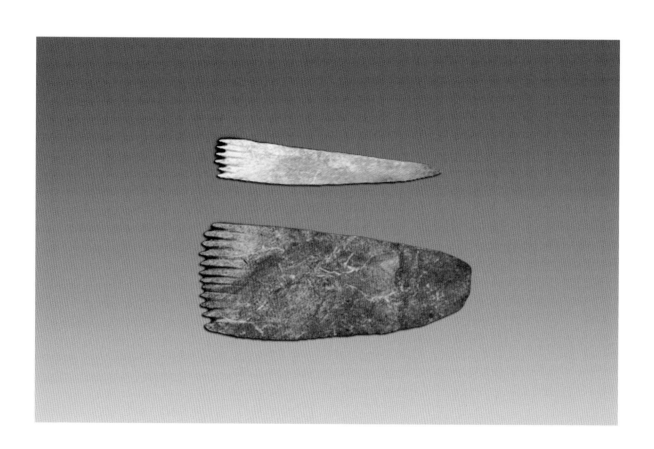

梳形器

新石器时代

骨质

上：长 8.5 厘米，宽 1.7 厘米

下：长 14 厘米，宽 13 厘米

Comb-shaped Articles

The Neolithic Age

Bone

Upper One: Length 8.5 cm/ Width 1.7 cm

Lower One: Length 14 cm/ Width 13 cm

梳形器两件，均以骨料切割磨制而成，一大一小。整体呈楔形，前宽后窄，宽的一端加工出梳形的齿。拉萨曲贡遗址出土。

西藏博物馆藏

The two comb-shaped articles, a big one and a small one, were made of ground bone. The whole body of each article is wedge shaped, with the teeth processed at the wider end. The artifacts were unearthed at Qugong Late Neolithic Site in Lhasa.

Preserved in Tibet Museum

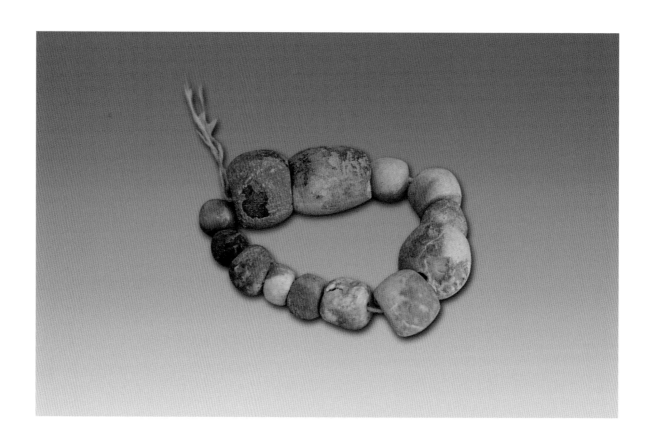

佩珠

新石器时代

石质

重 43.5 克

Beads

The Neolithic Age

Stone

Weight 43.5 g

形似算盘珠，大小不一，呈白色、红色或黑色，中部穿孔。装饰品。陕西省澄城县征集。

陕西医史博物馆藏

Shaped like abacus beads of various size, the beads are white, red or black with perforations. The beads, an article for decoration, were collected from Chengcheng County, Shaanxi Province.

Preserved in Shaanxi Museum of Medical History

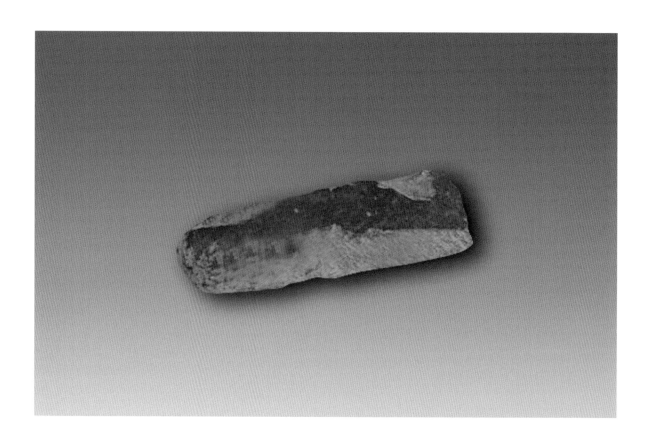

石斧

新石器时代

石质

长 11 厘米，宽 3.5 厘米，高 1.5 厘米，重 150 克

Stone Axe

The Neolithic Age

Stone

Length 11 cm/ Width 3.5 cm/ Height 1.5 cm/ Weight 150 g

斧状，表面较光滑，有残损。生活、生产工具。

陕西医史博物馆藏

The stone axe has a smooth surface but is
incomplete. It was used as a labor tool or a living
utensil.

Preserved in Shaanxi Museum of Medical History

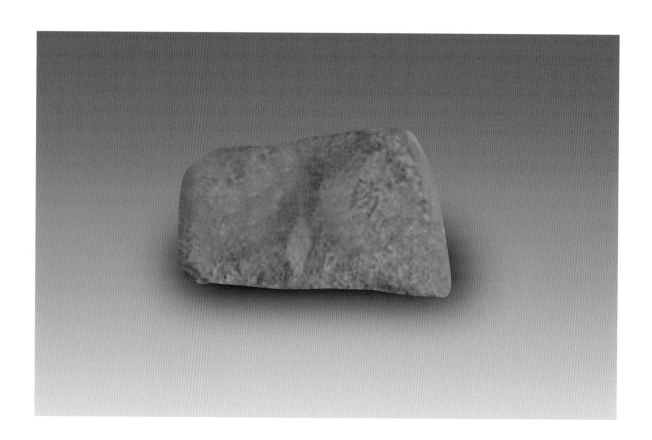

石斧

新石器时代

石质

长 9 厘米，宽 6 厘米，高 2 厘米，重 450 克

Stone Axe

The Neolithic Age

Stone

Length 9 cm/ Width 6 cm/ Height 2 cm/ Weight 450 g

斧状，边缘有残损。陕西省科学院（原中国
科学院陕西分院）上交。

陕西医史博物馆藏

The stone axe is hatchet-shaped and the edge
is incomplete. It was collected from Shaanxi
Academy of Sciences (former Shaanxi Branch
of Chinese Academy of Sciences).

Preserved in Shaanxi Museum of Medical History

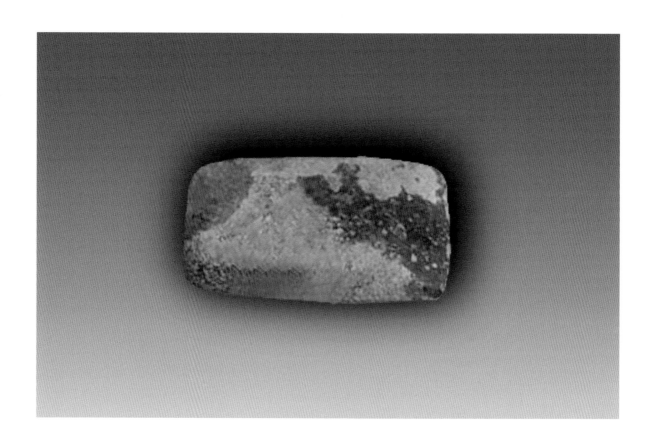

石斧

新石器时代

石质

长 10 厘米，宽 6 厘米，高 2 厘米，重 400 克

Stone Axe

The Neolithic Age

Stone

Length 10 cm/ Width 6 cm/ Height 2 cm/ Weight 400 g

斧状，边沿有残损。生产工具。陕西省西安
市东郊李家堡十里铺公社征集。

陕西医史博物馆藏

The stone axe is hatchet-shaped and the edge is incomplete. It was used as a labor tool. It was collected from Shilipu Commune of Lijiabu Village, which is located in the eastern suburb of Xi'an City, Shaanxi Province.

Preserved in Shaanxi Museum of Medical History

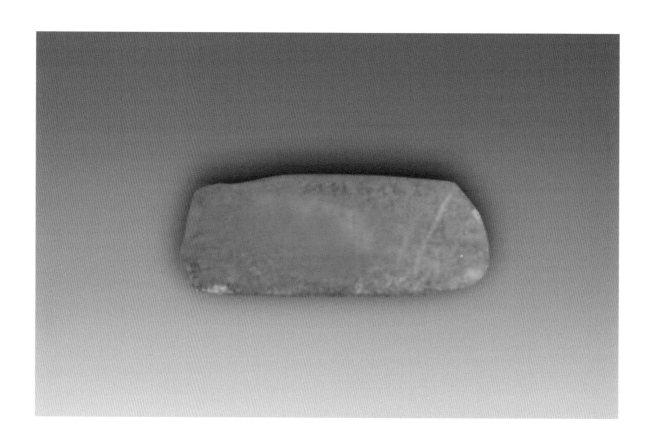

石斧

新石器时代

石质

长 13.5 厘米，宽 7 厘米，厚 0.8 厘米，重 350 克

Stone Axe

The Neolithic Age

Stone

Length 13.5 cm/ Width 7 cm/ Thickness 0.8 cm/ Weight 350 g

斧状，边沿有残损。生产工具。陕西省西安市蒋志坚老师捐赠。

陕西医史博物馆藏

The stone axe is hatchet-shaped and the edge is incomplete. It was used as a labor tool. It was donated by Jiang Zhijian, a teacher from Xi'an, Shaanxi Province.

Preserved in Shaanxi Museum of Medical History

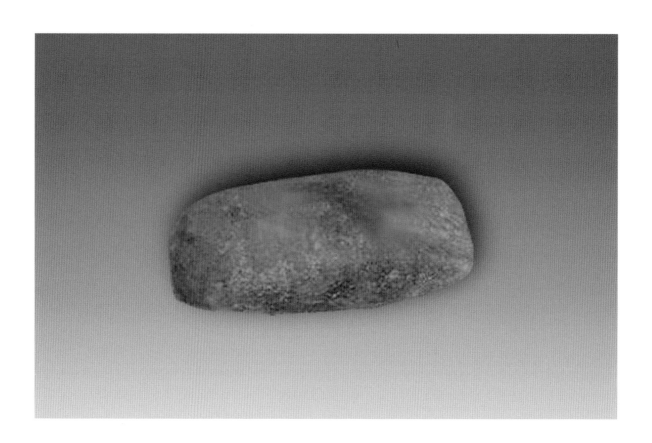

石斧

新石器时代

石质

长 14 厘米，通高 5.5 厘米，重 1010 克

Stone Axe

The Neolithic Age

Stone

Length 14 cm/ Height 5.5 cm/ Weight 1,010 g

斧状。生产工具。完整无损。

陕西医史博物馆藏

The hatchet-shaped stone axe was used as a labor tool. It is still in good condition.

Preserved in Shaanxi Museum of Medical History

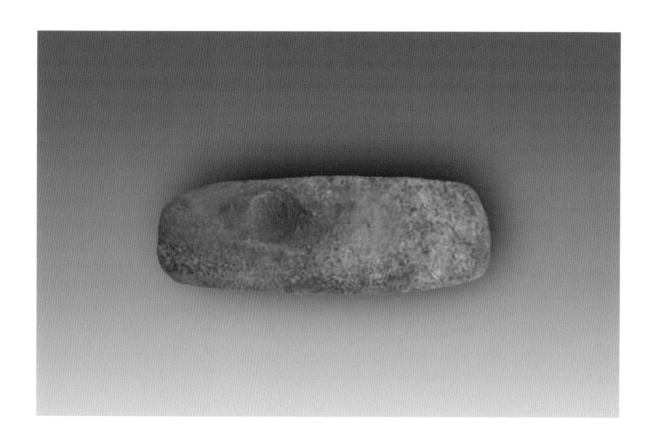

石斧

新石器时代

石质

长 8.5 厘米，宽 4 厘米，厚 1 厘米，重 48 克

Stone Axe

The Neolithic Age

Stone

Length 8.5 cm/ Width 4 cm/ Thickness 1 cm/ Weight 48 g

刀状，有残损。生产工具。陕西省西安市灞
桥征集。

陕西医史博物馆藏

The stone relic is shaped like a knife and is
incomplete. It was used as a labor tool. It was
collected from Baqiao District of Xi'an, Shaanxi
Province.

Preserved in Shaanxi Museum of Medical History

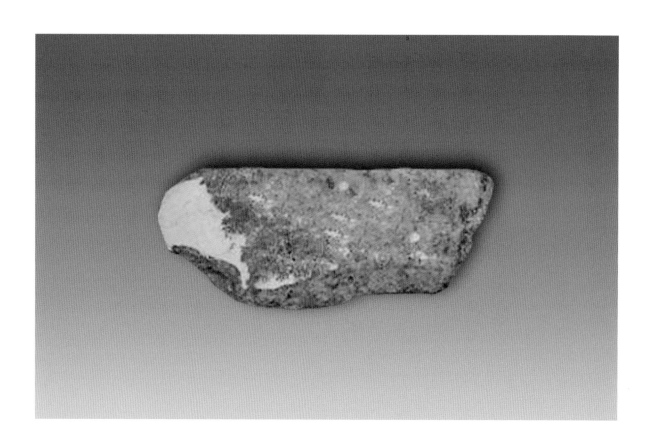

石斧

新石器时代

石质

长 10.5 厘米，宽 6 厘米，厚 2 厘米，重 250 克

Stone Axe

The Neolithic Age

Stone

Length 10.5 cm/ Width 6 cm/ Thickness 2 cm/ Weight 250 g

斧状。生产工具。完整无损。陕西省澄城县
征集。

陕西医史博物馆藏

The hatchet-shaped stone axe was used as a labor tool. It is still in good shape. It was collected from Chengcheng County, Shaanxi Province.

Preserved in Shaanxi Museum of Medical History

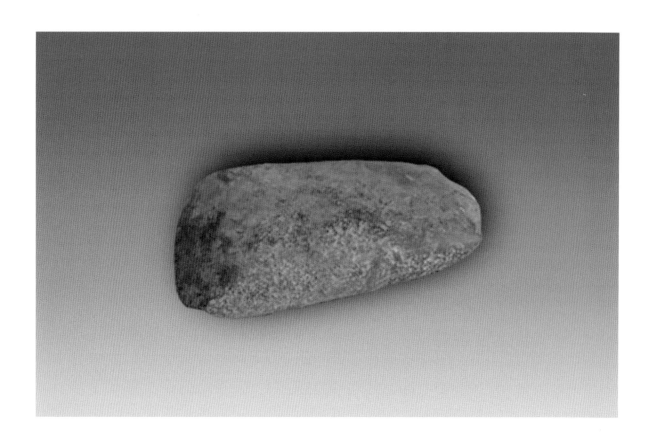

石铲

新石器时代

石质

长 17.5 厘米，宽 16 厘米，重 1050 克

Stone Shovel

The Neolithic Age

Stone

Length 17.5 cm/ Width 16 cm/ Weight 1,050 g

铲状。生产工具。完整无损。

陕西医史博物馆藏

The shovel-shaped stone relic was used as a labor tool. It is still in good condition.

Preserved in Shaanxi Museum of Medical History

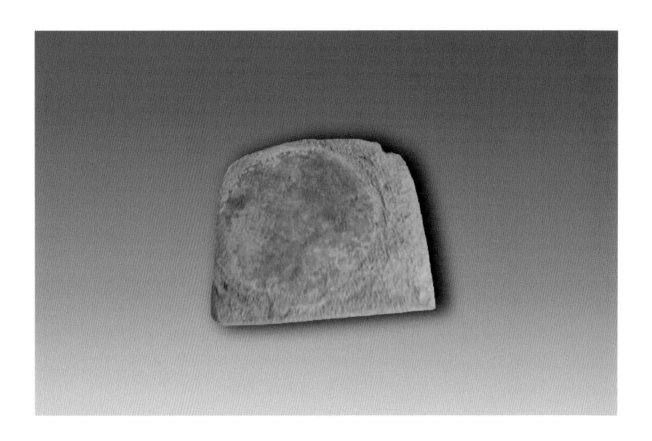

石铲

新石器时代

石质

长 17.5 厘米，宽 16 厘米，重 1050 克

Stone Shovel

The Neolithic Age

Stone

Length 17.5 cm/ Width 16 cm/ Weight 1,050 g

铲状。生产工具。完整无损。

陕西医史博物馆藏

The shovel-shaped stone relic was used as a labor tool. It is still in good condition.

Preserved in Shaanxi Museum of Medical History

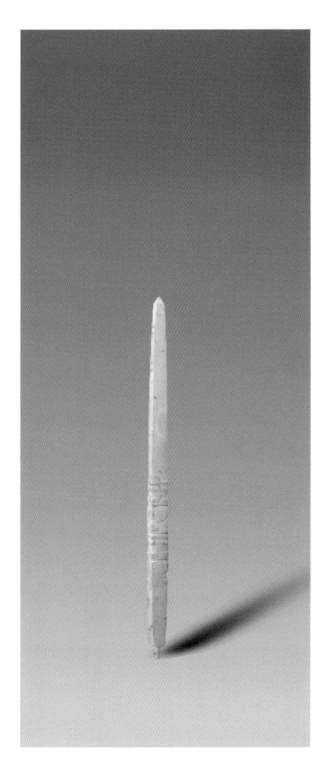

玉锥

新石器时代良渚文化

玉质

长 18.4 厘米

Jade Cone

Liangzhu Culture during Neolithic Age

Jade

Length 18.4 cm

器表呈白色，有透光的晶块。上半截呈圆锥形，下半截呈方柱形，以转角为中轴线，分为四节，每两节组合成神人兽面纹。下端琢成小短榫，并钻有横向小孔。在很小的方柱体上以浅浮雕和阴刻纹雕琢神徽图像，纹饰精细规整。

浙江省文物考古研究所藏

The cone has a white surface with transparent crystal blocks embedded. The upper part is cone-shaped. The lower part is shaped like a square column which has four sides with every two adjacent sides forming a section engraved with god-face, human-face, or beast-face mask. At the bottom is a short tenon with a horizontal drilling hole. On a small part of the square column surface engraved with fine bas-reliefs and elaborate intaglios of god emblem images. Preserved in Institute of Cultural Relics and Archaeology of Zhejiang Province

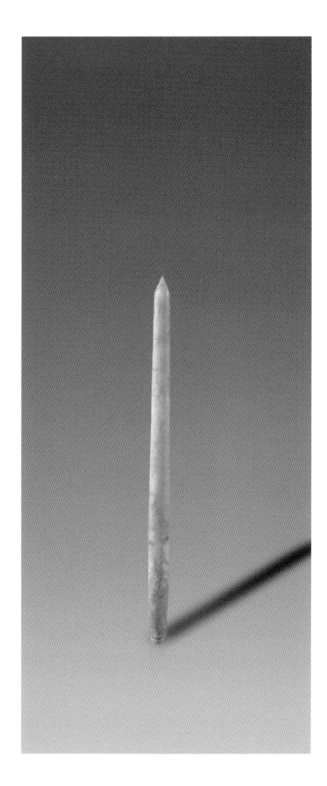

玉锥

新石器时代良渚文化

玉质

长 12.4 厘米

Jade Cone

Liangzhu Culture during Neolithic Age

Jade

Length 12.4 cm

白色玉，长圆锥形，一端尖锐，另一端有小
凸榫。器表琢磨光洁，制作精细。

常州博物馆藏

The piece of white jade is shaped like a slender
cone with a tip at one end and a small tenon at
the other. Its surface is finely and elaborately
polished.

Preserved in Changzhou Museum

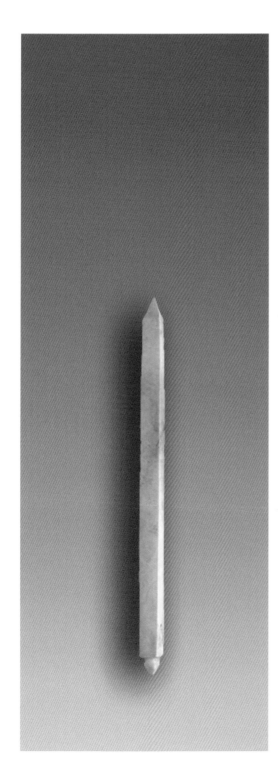

玉锥

新石器时代马桥文化

玉质

长 9.7 厘米

Jade Cone

Maqiao Culture during Neolithic Age

Jade

Length 9.7 cm

1997 年好川墓地出土。

遂昌县文物管理委员会藏

The cone was excavated at Haochuan Graveyard in 1997.
Preserved in the Cultural Relics Administration Committee of Suichang County

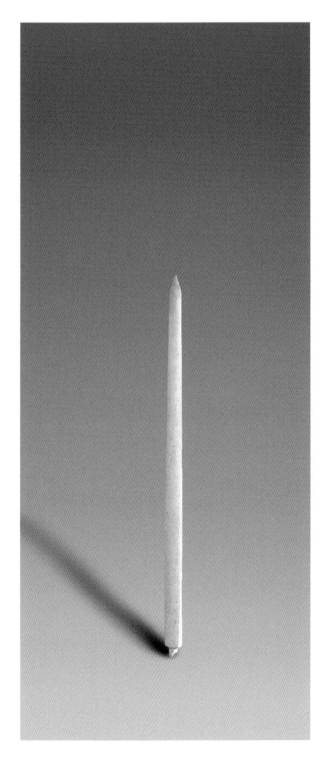

玉锥

新石器时代马桥文化

玉质

长 16.6 厘米

Jade Cone

Maqiao Culture during Neolithic Age

Jade

Length 16.6 cm

1997 年好川墓地出土。

遂昌县文物管理委员会藏

The cone was excavated at Haochuan Graveyard
in 1997.
Preserved in the Cultural Relics Administration
Committee of Suichang County

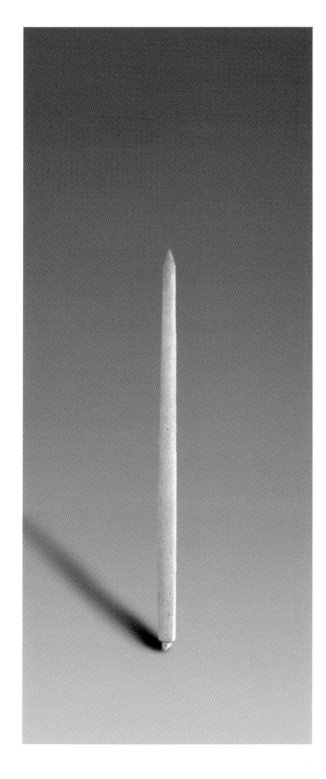

玉锥

新石器时代马桥文化

玉质

长 12 厘米

Jade Cone

Maqiao Culture during Neolithic Age

Jade

Length 12 cm

1997 年好川墓地出土。

遂昌县文物管理委员会藏

The cone was excavated at Haochuan Graveyard in 1997.

Preserved in the Cultural Relics Administration Committee of Suichang County

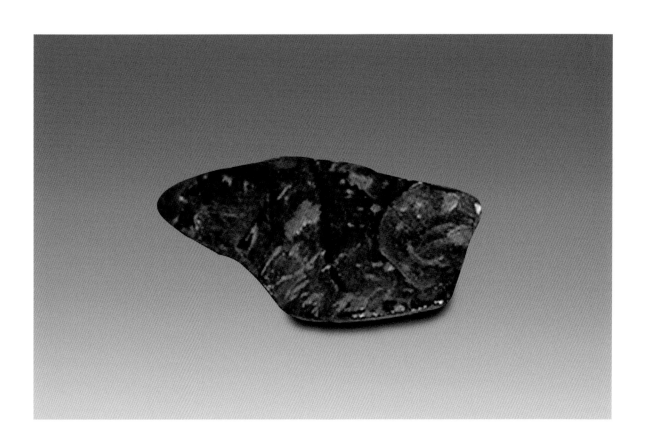

石砭

石器时代

石质

长约 4 厘米

Stone Medical Tool

The Stone Age

Stone

Length about 4 cm

不规则形，赭石色，一端打制成刃。医疗器
具。内蒙古博物院调拨。

陕西医史博物馆藏

The collection is irregular in shape and ochre-
colored. With one end made into blade, it was
utilized as a medical device. It was allocated
from Inner Mongolia Museum.

Preserved in Shaanxi Museum of Medical History

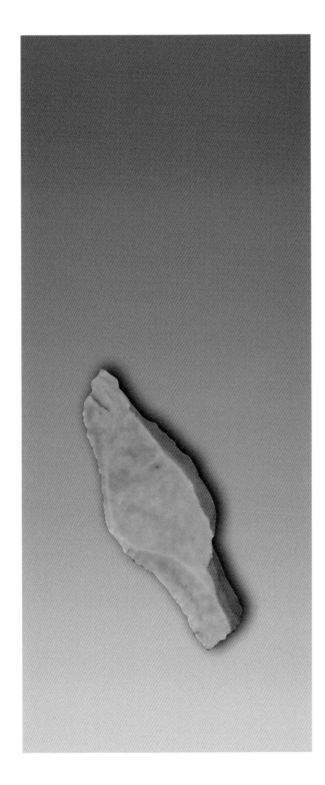

砭石

石器时代

石质

长 3.5 厘米，宽 1.3 厘米，厚 0.4 厘米

Stone Needle

The Stone Age

Stone

Length 3.5 cm/ Width 1.3 cm/ Thickness 0.4 cm

灰色硅质岩打制。镞尖状，两侧有刃，末端有梃。可用于放血、破痈。

　　中华医学会／上海中医药大学医史博物馆藏

The stone needle is made of gray siliceous rock and is arrowhead-shaped, with blade on both sides and iron ore at the tip. It was used for bloodletting and breaking carbuncles.

Preserved in Chinese Medical Association/ Museum of Chinese Medicine, Shanghai University of Traditional Chinese Medicine

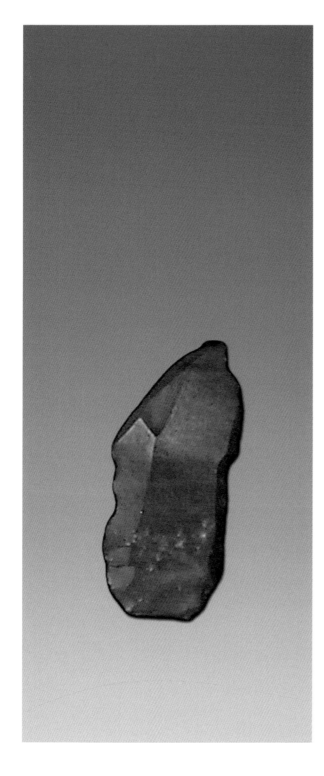

砭石

石器时代

石质

长 3 厘米，宽 1.2 厘米，厚 0.3 厘米

Stone Needle

The Stone Age

Stone

Length 3 cm/ Width 1.2 cm/ Thickness 0.3 cm

黄棕色硅质岩剥落的石叶加工而成。镞尖状，
两侧有刃，表面光滑。医用。

　　中华医学会 / 上海中医药大学医史博物馆藏

The stone needle is made of pieces of yellow
brown siliceous rock. It is arrowhead-shaped,
with blade on both sides and a smooth surface. It
was used for medical purposes.

Preserved in Chinese Medical Association/ Museum
of Chinese Medicine, Shanghai University of
Traditional Chinese Medicine

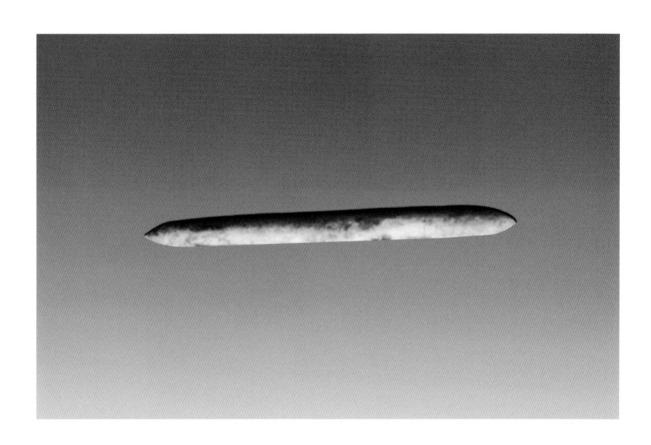

玉针

商

玉质

长 9.3 厘米，直径 0.39 厘米，重 6 克

Jade Pin

Shang Dynasty

Jade

Length 9.3 cm/ Diameter 0.39 cm/ Weight 6 g

白色细腻玉料磨制而成，近圆柱形，两端有

尖。可用于放血、破痈。

广东中医药博物馆藏

The pin, made of delicate white jade material by grinding, is nearly cylindrical but pointed at both ends. It was used for bloodletting and breaking carbuncles.

Preserved in Guangdong Chinese Medicine Museum

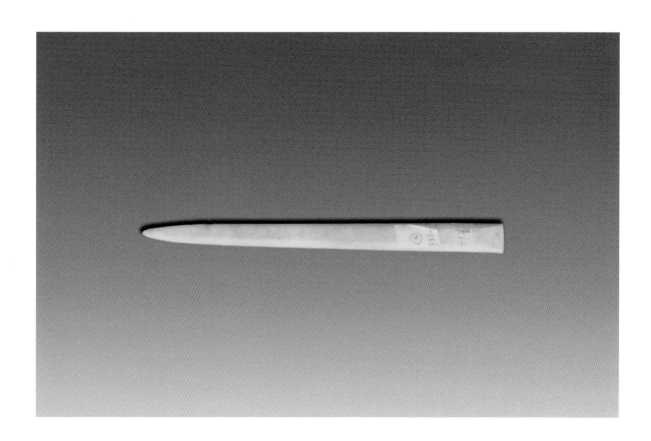

玉针

商

玉质

长 11.4 厘米，底宽 0.67 厘米，厚 0.14 厘米，重 8 克

Jade Pin

Shang Dynasty

Jade

Length 11.4 cm/ Bottom Width 0.67 cm/ Thickness 0.14 cm/ Weight 8 g

白色细腻玉料磨制而成，扁平锥形，一端有
尖，另一端平直。可用于放血、破痈。

广东中医药博物馆藏

The pin is made of delicate white jade material
by grinding. It is conical, pointed at one end
and flat at the other end. The pin was used for
bloodletting and breaking carbuncles.

Preserved in Guangdong Chinese Medicine Museum

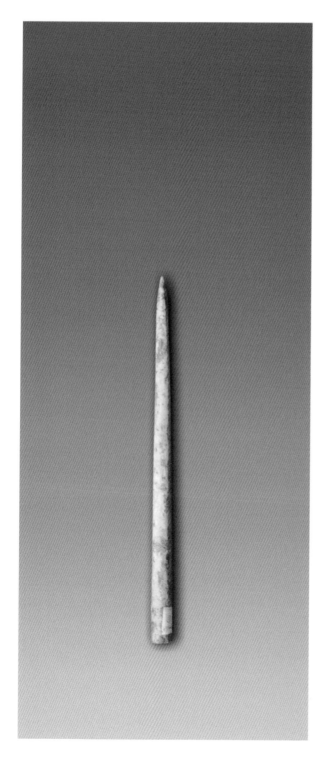

玉针

商

玉质

长 18.2 厘米，底部直径 0.78 厘米，重 17 克

Jade Pin

Shang Dynasty

Jade

Length 18.2 cm/ Bottom Diameter 0.78 cm/ Weight

17 g

青灰色细腻玉料磨制而成，圆锥形，一端有
尖，另一端较平。可用于放血、破痈。

广东中医药博物馆藏

The pin is made of delicate green gray jade
material by grinding. It is conical, pointed at one
end and flat at the other end. It was used for
bloodletting and breaking carbuncles.

Preserved in Guangdong Chinese Medicine Museum

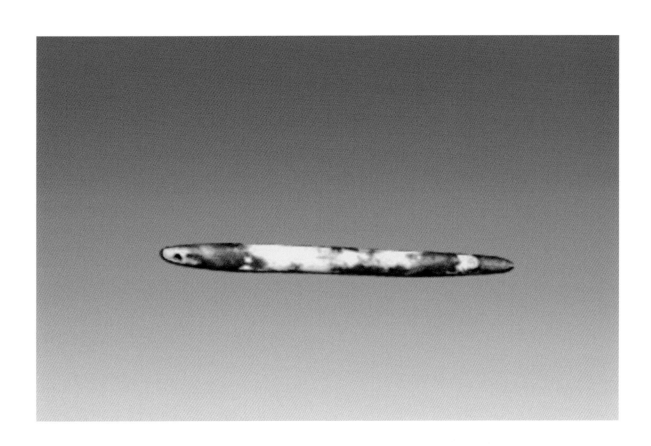

玉针

商

玉质

长 7.5 厘米，直径 0.62 厘米

Jade Pin

Shang Dynasty

Jade

Length 7.5 cm/ Diameter 0.62 cm

白色细腻玉料磨制而成，细长纺锤形，中间
粗，两端细，一端有尖，另一端穿孔。可用
于放血、破痈。

广东中医药博物馆藏

The pin is made of delicate white jade material
by grinding. It is elongated and spindle-shaped,
thick in the middle and thin on both ends.
One end is perforated. The pin was used for
bloodletting and breaking carbuncles.
Preserved in Guangdong Chinese Medicine Museum

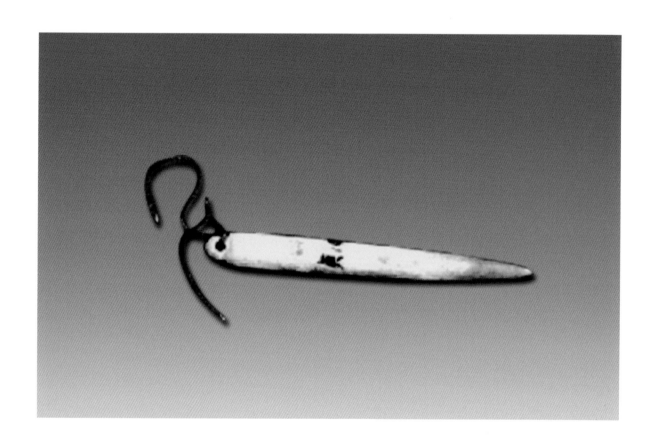

玉针

商

玉质

长 3.2 厘米，直径 0.47 厘米

Jade Pin

Shang Dynasty

Jade

Length 3.2 cm/ Diameter 0.47 cm

白色细腻玉料磨制而成，圆锥形，一端有尖，

另一端圆滑，有穿孔。可用于放血、破痈。

广东中医药博物馆藏

The pin was made of delicate white jade material

by grinding. It is conical, pointed at one end and

round at the other end, which is pierced. It was

used for bloodletting and breaking carbuncles.

Preserved in Guangdong Chinese Medicine Museum

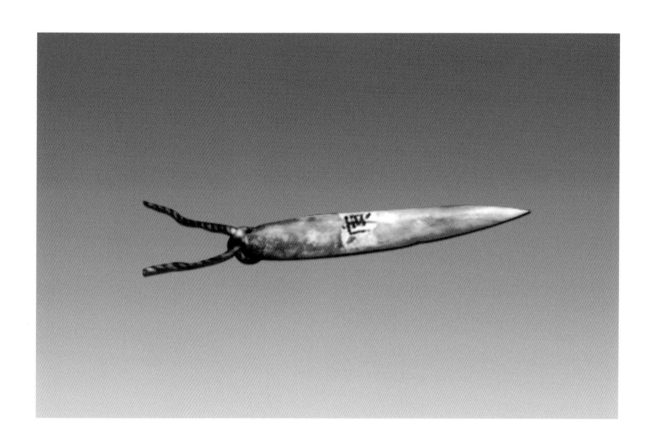

玉针

商

玉质

长 5.3 厘米，直径 0.5 厘米

Jade Pin

Shang Dynasty

Jade

Length 5.3 cm/ Diameter 0.5 cm

褐色细腻玉料磨制而成，圆锥形，一端有尖，

另一端圆滑，有穿孔。可用于放血、破痈。

广东中医药博物馆藏

The pin is made of delicate brown jade material
by grinding. It is conical, pointed at one end
and round at the other end, which is perforated.
The pin was used for bloodletting and breaking
carbuncles.

Preserved in Guangdong Chinese Medicine Museum

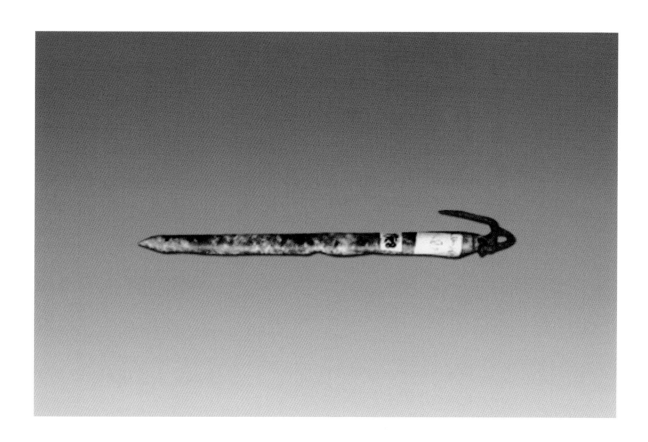

玉针

商

玉质

长 10.2 厘米，直径 0.37 厘米

Jade Pin

Shang Dynasty

Jade

Length 10.2 cm/ Diameter 0.37 cm

褐色细腻玉料磨制而成，圆锥形，一端有尖，

另一端圆滑，有穿孔。可用于放血、破痈。

广东中医药博物馆藏

The pin is made of delicate brown jade material by grinding. It is conical, pointed at one end and round at the other end, which is perforated. The pin was used for bloodletting and breaking carbuncles.

Preserved in Guangdong Chinese Medicine Museum

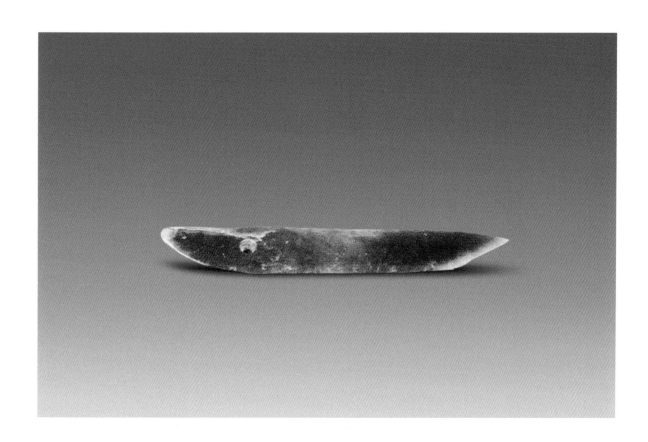

玉刀

商

玉质

长 10.5 厘米

Jade Carving Knife

Shang Dynasty

Jade

Length 10.5 cm

褐色细腻玉料磨制而成，形似璋，两端皆尖，

一端有刃，一端穿孔。可用作手术刀，亦可

用作原始的医疗活动。

上海中医药博物馆藏

The knife is made of delicate brown jade
material by grinding. It is shaped like a flat
rectangle, but pointed at both ends. There is
blade at one end and a perforation at the other
end. It was used either as a carving knife or for
primitive medical activities.

Preserved in Shanghai Museum of Traditional
Chinese Medicine

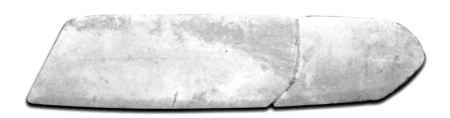

玉刀

商

玉质

长 18.3 厘米，宽 4.6 厘米，重 115 克

Jade Knife

Shang Dynasty

Jade

Length 18.3 cm/ Width 4.6 cm/ Weight 115 g

青色细腻玉料磨制而成，形似璋，器身扁薄，

直背，直刃略凸，一端有尖，另一端较圆滑。

工具、礼器，或用于医疗排脓、放血。

广东中医药博物馆藏

The sword is made of delicate cyan jade material by grinding. It has a thin body, a vertical back, and a slightly convex edge. It is pointed at one end and smooth at the other end. The sword was used as a tool or a sacrificial vessel, or for draining abscess and bloodletting.

Preserved in Guangdong Chinese Medicine Museum

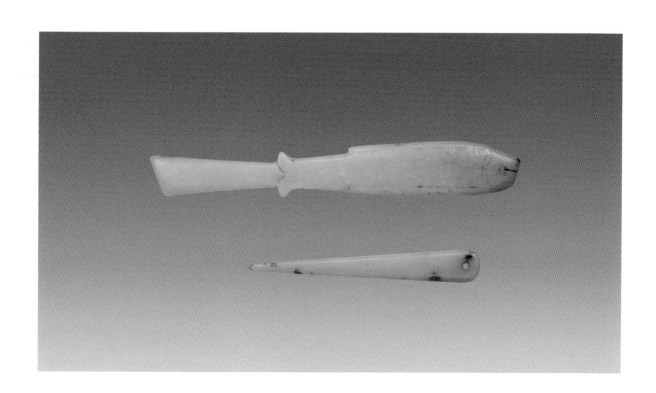

玉质针刀

商

玉质

上：长 13.3 厘米，宽 1.7 厘米

下：长 8.2 厘米，宽 0.9 厘米

Jade Needle-knives

Shang Dynasty

Jade

Upper One: Length 13.3 cm/ Width 1.7 cm

Lower One: Length 8.2 cm/ Width 0.9 cm

此两件针刀玉质相同，通体磨制而成，做工精巧细致。一枚为刀具，鱼形柄，梯形刃，柄首有穿孔，与殷墟古墓出土的鱼形扁状器类似。另一枚为针具，呈狭长的三角形，首部也有穿孔，用于穴位按压。

张雅宗藏

The two needle-knives, ground out of whole jade piece of the same quality, show exquisite workmanship. One is a knife with a fish-shaped handle, a trapezoid blade and a hole on the head of the handle. It resembles flat fish-shaped artifacts unearthed from ancient tombs in Yin Dynasty Ruins. The other is a narrow and long triangular needle with a hole on its top. It was used for pressing acupoints.

Collected by Zhang Yazong

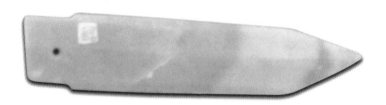

玉戈

商

玉质

长 6.8 厘米，宽 1.2 厘米，厚 0.36 厘米，重 3.3 克

Jade Dagger-axe

Shang Dynasty

Jade

Length 6.8 cm/ Width 1.2 cm/ Thickness 0.36 cm/ Weight 3.3 g

褐色细腻玉料磨制而成，形似圭，器身扁薄，

一端有尖，另一端有肩，且钻孔。两侧有刃，

中部有脊。兵器、礼器，或用于医疗排脓、

放血。

广东中医药博物馆藏

The jade dagger-axe is made of delicate brown jade material by grinding. It is shaped like a thin rectangle. It is pointed at one end and perforated at the other. There is blade on both sides and a ridge in the middle. It was used as a weapon or a sacrificial vessel, or for draining abscess and bloodletting.

Preserved in Guangdong Chinese Medicine Museum

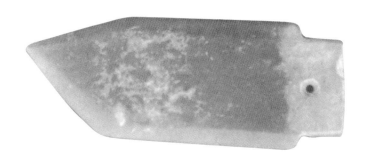

玉戈

商

玉质

长 4.3 厘米，宽 1.6 厘米，厚 0.21 厘米，重 3.35 克

Jade Dagger-axe

Shang Dynasty

Jade

Length 4.3 cm/ Width 1.6 cm/ Thickness 0.21 cm/ Weight 3.35 g

褐色细腻玉料磨制而成，形似圭，器身扁薄，

一端有尖，另一端有肩，且钻孔。两侧有刃。

兵器、礼器，或用于医疗排脓、放血。

广东中医药博物馆藏

The jade dagger-axe is made of delicate brown jade material by grinding. It is shaped like a flat rectangle. It is pointed at one end and there are a shoulder and a perforation at the other end. Both sides of the jade dagger-axe are edged. It was used as a weapon or a sacrificial vessel, or for draining abscess and bloodletting.

Preserved in Guangdong Chinese Medicine Museum

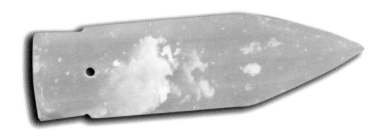

玉戈

商

玉质

长 7 厘米，最宽 2.2 厘米，厚 0.2 厘米，重 7.9 克

Jade Dagger-axe

Shang Dynasty

Jade

Length 7 cm/ Maximum Width 2.2 cm/ Thickness 0.2 cm/ Weight 7.9 g

褐色细腻玉料磨制而成，形似圭，器身扁薄，

一端有尖，另一端有肩，且钻孔。两侧有刃，

中部有脊。兵器、礼器，或用于医疗排脓、

放血。

广东中医药博物馆藏

The jade dagger-axe is made of delicate brown jade material by grinding. It is a flat rectangle with a thin body. It is pointed at one end and has a shoulder and a perforation at the other end. Both sides of the jade dagger-axe are edged and the central part has a ridge. It was used as a weapon or a sacrificial vessel, or for draining abscess and bloodletting.

Preserved in Guangdong Chinese Medicine Museum

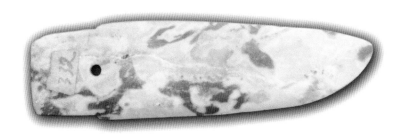

玉戈

商

玉质

长 10.4 厘米，最宽 3 厘米，厚 0.4 厘米，重 25 克

Jade Dagger-axe

Shang Dynasty

Jade

Length 10.4 cm/ Maximum Width 3 cm/ Thickness 0.4 cm/ Weight 25 g

黑白相间的细腻玉料磨制而成，形似圭，器身扁薄，一端有尖，另一端有肩，且钻孔。两侧有刃。兵器、礼器，或用于医疗排脓、放血。

广东中医药博物馆藏

The jade dagger-axe is made of black and white delicate jade material by grinding. It is a flat rectangle with a thin body. It is pointed at one end and has a shoulder and a perforation at the other end. Both sides of the jade dagger-axe are edged. It was used as a weapon or a sacrificial vessel, or for draining abscess and bloodletting.

Preserved in Guangdong Chinese Medicine Museum

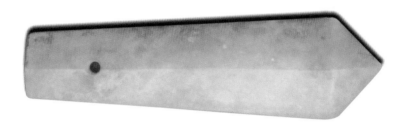

玉戈

商

玉质

长 14.5 厘米，最宽 4.3 厘米，厚 0.29 厘米，穿孔距斧刃 11.3 厘米，重 55 克

Jade Dagger-axe

Shang Dynasty

Jade

Length 14.5 cm/ Maximum Width 4.3 cm/ Thickness 0.29 cm/ Perforation to Axe Blade 11.3 cm/ Weight 55 g

青色细腻玉料磨制而成，形似圭，器身扁薄，

一端有尖，另一端较平，且钻孔。两侧有刃，

中部有脊。兵器、礼器，或用于医疗排脓、

放血。

广东中医药博物馆藏

The jade dagger-axe is made of delicate cyan jade material by grinding. It is a flat rectangle with a thin body. It is pointed at one end and has a shoulder and a perforation at the other end. Both sides of the jade dagger-axe are edged and the central part has a ridge. It was used as a weapon or a sacrificial vessel, or for draining abscess and bloodletting.

Preserved in Guangdong Chinese Medicine Museum

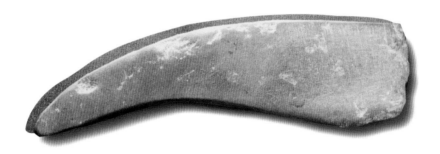

砭镰

商

石质

长 20 厘米，最宽 5.4 厘米

Stone Sickle

Shang Dynasty

Stone

Length 20 cm/ Maximum Width 5.4 cm

通体磨制而成，形似镰刀，一端粗，一端细。

1973 年河北藁城台西村商代第 14 号墓出土，

出土时置于一漆盒内。经考证系当时的医疗

用具。

河北省文物研究所藏

The whole sickle is made by grinding. It is shaped like a sickle, thick at one end and thin at the other end. The sickle was excavated in a lacquered box at Shang Dynasty Tomb No. 14 in Taixi Village in Haocheng, Hebei Province, in 1973. Based on textual research, it has been confirmed to have been used as a medical tool.

Preserved in Cultural Relics Institute of Hebei Province

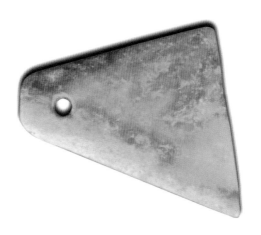

玉斧

商

玉质

长边 7 厘米，短边 6 厘米，刃宽 5.5 厘米，穿孔距斧刃 4.4 厘米，重 28 克

Jade Axe

Shang Dynasty

Jade

Maximum Length 7 cm/ Minimum Length 6 cm/ Blade Width 5.5 cm/ Perforation to Axe Blade 4.4 cm/ Weight 28 g

青灰色细腻玉料磨制而成，器身扁薄，刃部宽大，首部较圆滑，且有一穿孔。生产工具、兵器或礼器，也可用于医疗。

广东中医药博物馆藏

The axe is made of greenish gray delicate jade material by grinding. It has a thin body, a broad blade, a smooth head, and a perforation. The axe was used as a tool of production, a weapon or a sacrificial tool, or for medical treatment.

Preserved in Guangdong Chinese Medicine Museum

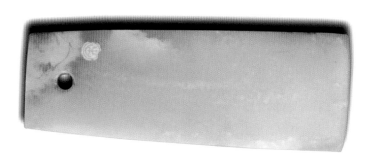

玉斧

商

玉质

长 13.6 厘米，宽 4.6 厘米，厚 0.49 厘米，穿孔距斧刃 11.5 厘米，重 133 克

Jade Axe

Shang Dynasty

Jade

Length 13.6 cm/ Width 4.6 cm/ Thickness 0.49 cm/ Perforation to Axe Blade 11.5 cm/ Weight 133 g

青色细腻玉料磨制而成，器身扁薄，近梯形，刃部较宽，首部有一钻孔。生产工具、兵器或礼器，也可用于医疗。

广东中医药博物馆藏

The axe is made of delicate cyan jade material by grinding. Shaped trapezoidal, it has a flat and thin body, a broad blade, and a perforated head. The axe was used as a tool of production, a weapon or a sacrificial tool, or for medical treatment.

Preserved in Guangdong Chinese Medicine Museum

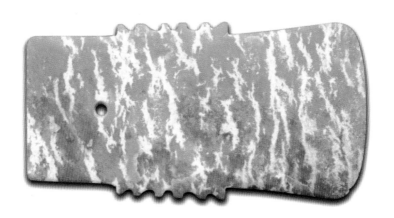

玉斧

商

玉质

长 16.8 厘米，宽 8 厘米，厚 0.49 厘米，穿孔距斧刃 13.8 厘米，重 175 克

Jade Axe

Shang Dynasty

Jade

Length 16.8 cm/ Width 8 cm/ Thickness 0.49 cm/ Perforation to Axe Blade 13.8 cm/ Weight 175 g

青色细腻玉料磨制而成，器身扁薄，近梯形，刃部呈弧形，两端上翘。首部有肩，中部钻孔。斧身两侧边各有 6 个棘突，对称分布。生产工具、兵器或礼器，也可用于医疗。

广东中医药博物馆藏

The axe is made of delicate cyan jade material by grinding. Shaped trapezoidal, it has a flat and thin body, a curved blade, and two cocking-up ends. And there is a shoulder on its head and a perforation in its central part. Both sides of the axe body have six spinous processes which are symmetrically distributed. The axe was used as a tool of production, a weapon or a sacrificial tool, or for medical treatment.

Preserved in Guangdong Chinese Medicine Museum

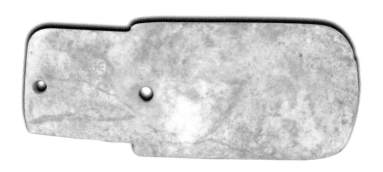

石斧

商

石质

通长 12.5 厘米，最宽 5.3 厘米，最窄 4 厘米，两穿孔分别距斧刃 7.6 厘米和 12 厘米，重 130 克

Stone Axe

Shang Dynasty

Stone

Length 12.5 cm/ Maximum Width 5.3 cm/ Minimum Width 4 cm/ Perforation to Axe Blade 7.6 cm and 12 cm/ Weight 130 g

通体磨制而成，器身扁薄，近方形，刃部呈
弧形。首部有肩，肩中部和首端各有一钻孔。
生产工具、兵器或礼器，也可用于医疗。

广东中医药博物馆藏

The axe is made by grinding. It is nearly square
with a thin body and curved blades. The axe
has a shoulder on its head; there is a perforation
in both the middle part of the shoulder and the
head. The axe was used as a tool of production,
a weapon or a sacrificial tool, or for medical
treatment.

Preserved in Guangdong Chinese Medicine Museum

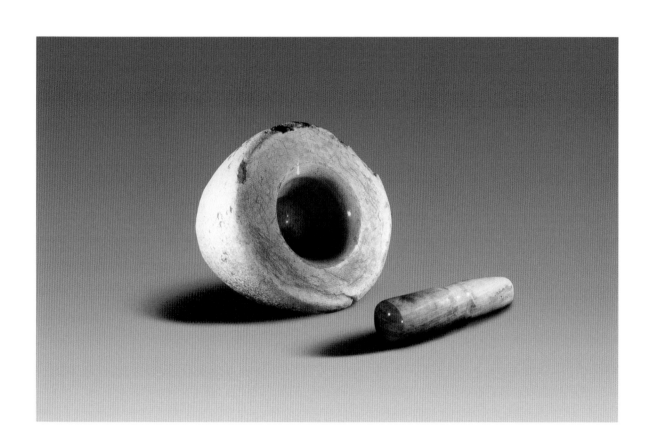

玉臼、玉杵

商

玉质

臼：高 23.2 厘米，口径 29.5 厘米，孔径 16 厘米，深
13 厘米，壁厚 8 厘米

杵：长 28 厘米

Jade Mortar and Pestle

Shang Dynasty

Jade

Mortar: Height 23.2 cm/ Mouth Diameter
29.5 cm/ Hole Diameter 16 cm/ Depth 13 cm/
Wall Thickness 8 cm

Pestle: Length 28 cm

细腻玉料磨制而成。臼敞口，壁较厚，臼孔
周壁有朱红色，鉴定为朱砂残迹。杵为棕色，
圆柱形，有使用痕迹。当为研药器具，朱砂
既可作颜料，亦可用作药物。1976 年河南省
安阳市殷墟妇好墓出土。

殷墟博物馆藏

The mortar and the pestle are made of delicate
jade material by grinding. The mortar has an
open mouth and thick wall. Around the wall
of the aperture is vermilion color, which has
been identified to be remnants of cinnabar,
which could be used as pigment and drug. The
brown and cylindrical pestle shows some traces
of using. The mortar and the pestle were utilized
for porphyrizing drug ingredients. The collection
was excavated from Fuhao's tomb in Yinxu of
Anyang City, Henan Province, in 1976.
Preserved in Yinxu Museum

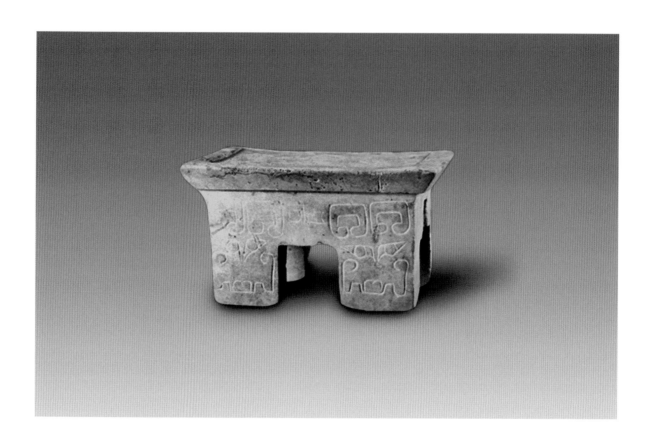

石俎

商

石质

长 22.7 厘米，宽 13.3 厘米，高 12.8 厘米

Stone Chopping Block

Shang Dynasty

Stone

Length 22.7 cm/ Width 13.3 cm/ Height 12.8 cm

此件形似现代的案几，以质料较纯的灰白色
石料制作而成，素雅洁净，与简洁的装饰气
氛十分谐调。俎在古代用于切割生肉并盛放
熟肉的器具，兼有今之砧板和托盘的功能。
还用于祭祀。河南省安阳市大司空出土。

北京大学赛克勒考古与艺术博物馆藏

This artifact, is made of grayish white stone
material with relative purity. Looking elegant
and clean, it matches the simple decoration
perfectly. The stone chopping block was an
ancient utensil used to chop raw meat and hole
cooked meat. It served as both a chopping block
and a tray. it was also utilized as a sacrificial
tool. It was unearthed in Dasikong of Anyang
City, Henan Province.
Preserved in Arthur M.Sackler Museum of Art
and Archaeology at Peking University

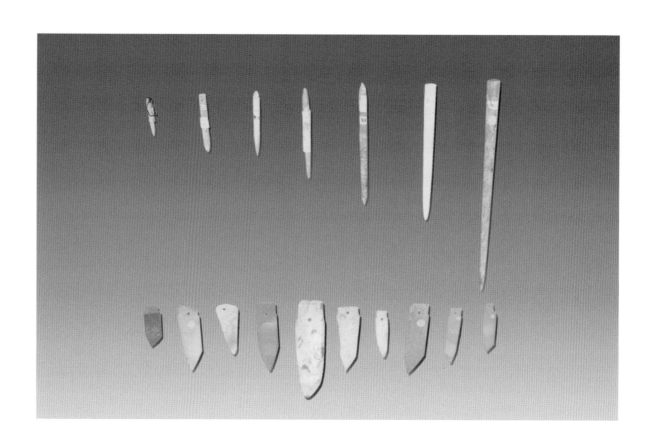

砭石、玉石针

商周

玉、石质

砭石：最长 6.2 厘米，最短 1.7 厘米

玉石针：最长 18 厘米，最短 2.5 厘米

Stone Needles and Jade Pins

Shang Dynasty and Zhou Dynasty

Jade and stone

Stone needles: Length 1.7–6.2 cm

Jade pins: Length 2.5–18 cm

该藏为砭石和玉石针各一组，皆用细腻的石料或玉料磨制而成。玉石针皆为锥状，一端尖锐，另一端多有穿孔。砭石皆为圭形，末端均有穿孔。

广东中医药博物馆藏

The group of stone needles and the group of jade pins are made of delicate stone or jade by grinding. The jade pins are awl-shaped, pointed at one end and perforated at the other end. The stone needles are nearly rectangular with a perforation at one end.

Preserved in Guangdong Chinese Medicine Museum

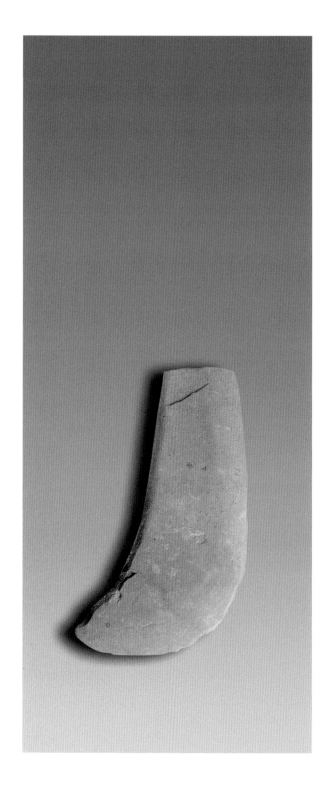

靴形石刀

商周

石质

长约 15 厘米

Boot-shaped Stone Knife

Shang Dynasty and Zhou Dynasty

Stone

Length about 15 cm

青灰色砂岩通体磨制而成，形似靴，凹背凸刃，刀尖上翘。为工具，也可作为医疗用具。

象山县文物管理委员会藏

The knife is made of greenish gray sandstone by grinding. Shaped like a boot, it has a concave back and a convex blade, with the point tilting upwards. It was used as a working tool or a medical tool.

Preserved in Xiangshan County Administration Committee of Cultural Relics

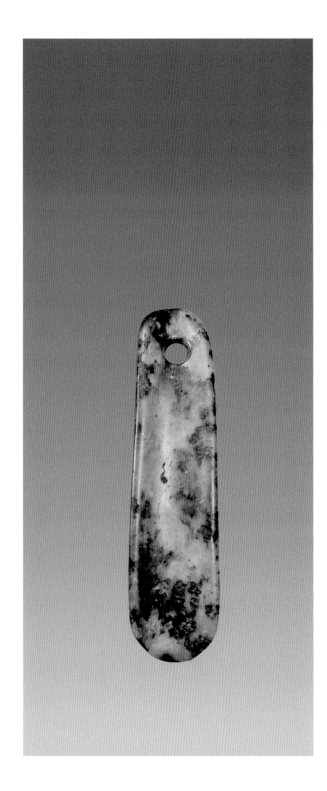

玉质异型刀

西周

玉质

长 6 厘米，宽 1.6 厘米

Irregular Jade Knife

Western Zhou Dynasty

Jade

Length 6 cm/ Width 1.6 cm

近狭长的长方形，系用细腻玉料通体磨制而成，一端有穿孔，另一端圆弧形，有刃。主要用于先民的简单外科手术，如去鸡眼，破除疖子和痈等。此类刀具出现时间较早，西周后期逐渐绝迹。

张雅宗藏

The long and narrow rectangular knife was ground out of fine whole jade material. It has a hole on one end and is shaped like an arc on the other. It was mainly used by primitive people in simple operations such as removing corns and carbuncles and piercing furuncles. This type of knife was invented in very early time but gradually disappeared in late Western Zhou Dynasty.

Collected by Zhang Yazong

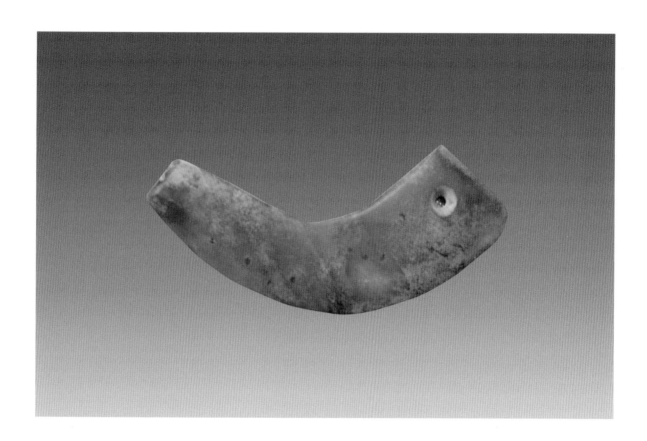

玉质异型刀

西周

玉质

长 7 厘米，宽 0.6 ~ 1.9 厘米

Irregular Jade Knife

Western Zhou Dynasty

Jade

Length 7 cm/ Width 0.6-1.9 cm

近镰刀形，系用细腻玉料通体磨制而成，一端有穿孔，边缘有刃。外形精巧，具有明显的医用特征。经中医医史研究专家鉴定后认为，出现如此异形玉质医用刀很可能是当时某小部族地区游医所配用的随身应急刀具，非中原地区之物。

张雅宗藏

The nearly sickle-shaped knife was ground out of fine whole jade material. There is a hole on one end and a blade on the edge. The delicate appearance suggests that it was obviously used for medical purpose. Experts of Traditional Chinese Medicine history concluded that this irregularly shaped jade knife, which did not originate from Central China, was very probably a tool carried by a roving doctor of a local tribe for emergency use.

Collected by Zhang Yazong

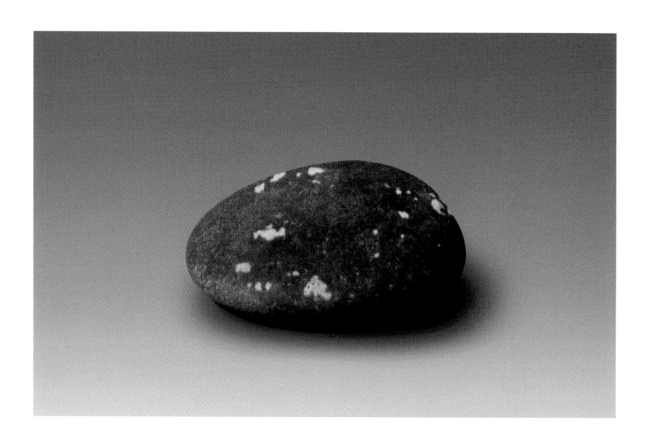

熨石

西周

石质

直径 6.5 厘米

Hotfix Stone

Western Zhou Dynasty

Stone

Diameter 6.5 cm

不规则红褐色扁圆石子。可用于熨治疾患。

陕西省扶风县周原召陈西周遗址出土。

宝鸡市周原博物馆藏

The stone, which is irregular, oval and reddish-brown, was used to treat diseases by ironing. It was excavated at Zhouyuan Zhaochen Site of the Western Zhou Dynasty, Fufeng County, Shaanxi Province.

Preserved in Zhouyuan Museum of Baoji City

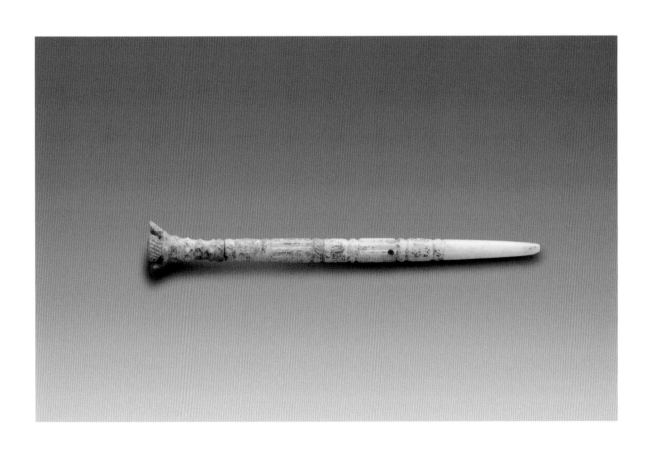

玉簪

春秋时代

玉质

长 16.2 厘米

Jade Hairpin

Spring and Autumn Period

Jade

Length 16.2 cm

白色细腻玉料磨制而成。分簪帽和簪身两部分，簪帽呈螺钉形，上粗下细，顶面中部下凹，上端雕琢纲纹，中部为乳丁纹，下部为绚索纹。簪身呈圆锥状，琢三组变形云纹和二组凹棱纹，每组之间隔以绚索纹，纹饰十分精细。簪身中部钻有一孔。器身局部受沁呈铁红色。全器打磨光滑，质地晶莹。为玉中之佳品。用以绾定发髻或冠。

南京市博物馆藏

The hairpin is made of white fine jade material by grinding. It consists of the cap and the body. The screw-shaped cap tapers downwards. The center of the top is slightly dented. The upper part is carved with nipple pattern; the middle part is carved with nipple pattern; the under part is carved with twisted cord design. The cone-shaped hairpin body is decorated with three groups of stylized cloud pattern and two groups of concave ribs, which are interspersed with twisted cord lines. A hole is drilled in the middle of the hairpin. Some parts of the body are oozed with iron red. This artifact is smooth and translucent. It was a treasure of jade for fixing bun or crown.

Preserved in Nanjing Municipal Museum

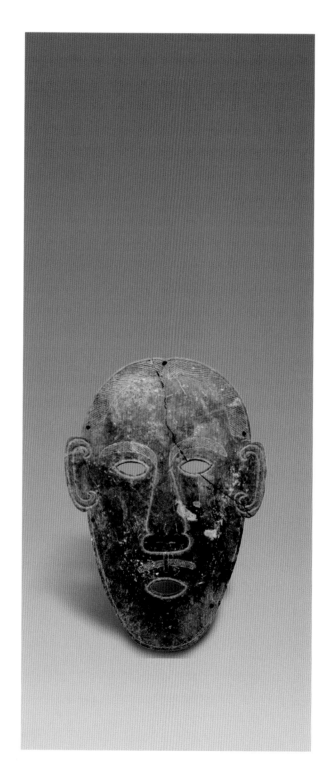

玉面罩

战国时代

玉质

长 20 厘米，宽 13.9 厘米，厚 0.23 厘米

Jade Mask

Warring States Period

Jade

Length 20 cm/ Width 13.9 cm/ Thickness 0.23 cm

为青色玉料制成。人物双眼及口镂空，耳、鼻、眉、须发均用细线阴刻，并且突出表现了鼻孔和人中。该面罩制作细致，说明当时人类对解剖学和人体的比例已经有了一定程度的掌握。

荆州博物馆藏

The mask, which is made of cyan jade material, has ears, nose, eyebrows and beard that were all incised with fine lines. It also has hollow-out eyes and mouth and highlights the nostrils and philtrum. The exquisite craftmanship of the mask shows that people at that time had achieved some mastery of anatomy and proportion of the human body.

Preserved in Jingzhou Museum

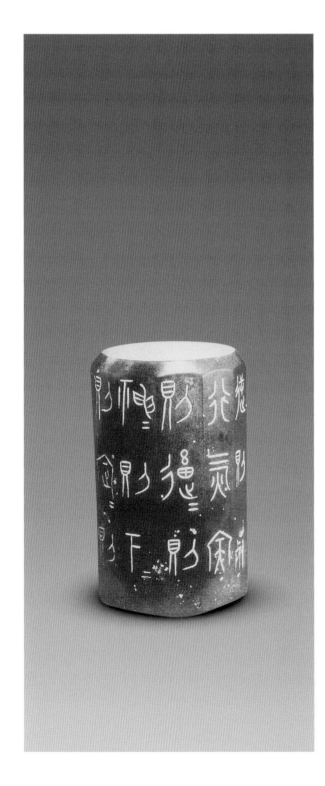

《行气铭》玉杖首

战国时代

玉质

底径 3.4 厘米，高 5.2 厘米

Jade Cane Head with Inscriptions about Circulation of Qi

Warring States Period

Jade

Bottom Diameter 3.4 cm/ Height 5.2 cm

玉制。呈十二面棱柱体，中空。在十二面中，每面竖刻三字，并有重文符号八个，共四十五字铭，扼要地讲述了行气的要领、过程和作用，是目前我们所见到的较早的关于行气理论的叙述。

天津博物馆藏

The cane head is a hollow and twelve-sided prism. Three words and eight repetitious passage symbols were incised on each side. The forty-five inscriptions briefly explain the key points, process and functions of promoting the circulation of Qi. It was an earlier narration of the theory of Qi circulation.

Preserved in Tianjin Museum

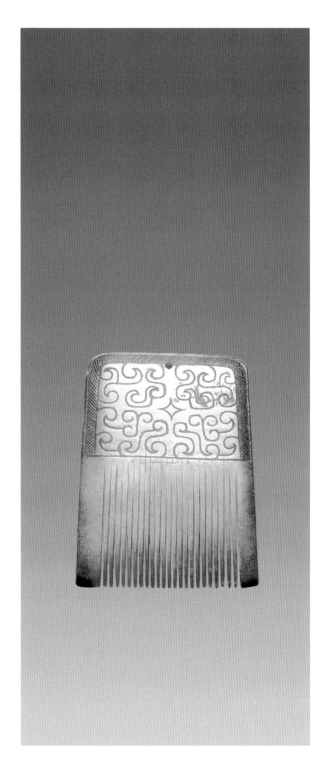

玉梳

战国时代

玉质

长 9.6 厘米，齿口宽 6.5 厘米，梳背宽 6 厘米

Jade Comb

Warring States Period

Jade

Length 9.6 cm/ Tooth Width 6.5 cm/ Back Width

6 cm

由白色玉料磨制而成。器形扁薄，梳齿修长
细密，梳背上细线阴刻卷云纹和斜线纹。造
型规整，表面光滑，工艺细致。

湖北省博物馆藏

The flat and thin comb is made of white jade
material by grinding. Its teeth are narrow and
slender; on the back of the comb is incised
cirrus clouds designs and diagonal lines. The
comb has structured modeling and smooth
surface and shows meticulous workmanship.
Preserved in Hubei Provincial Museum

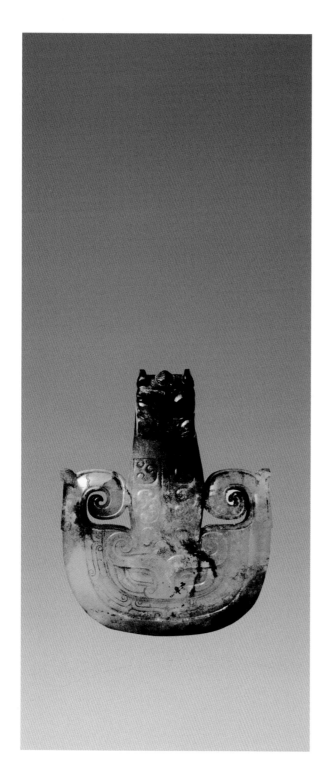

兽面纹玉带钩

战国时代

玉质

长 8.3 厘米，宽 6.8 厘米

Jade Belt Hook with Animal-faced Patterns

Warring States Period

Jade

Length 8.3 cm/ Width 6.8 cm

玉质晶莹，呈黄色。铲形，钩身饰兽面纹，双眼凸出，长眉上卷，左右及脊背阴刻出卷曲纹、花形纹、卷云纹等；钩端呈回首兽状。背面圆形钮，饰勾云纹等。形制特殊，雕刻精巧。

曲阜市文物局藏

This shovel-shaped hook is made of moisturized yellow jade. Its body is carved with an animal's face with protruded eyes and raised long eyebrows. Its left and right sides as well as its back are decorated with curled patterns, flower patterns and cirrus clouds in dented lines. The two ends of the hook look like two beast's, heads looking back. The back of the hook with a round knob is designed with diamond-shaped patterns and scrolled cloud patterns. The hook shows special design and shape and exquisite curving work.

Preserved in Qufu Municipal Bureau of Cultural Relics

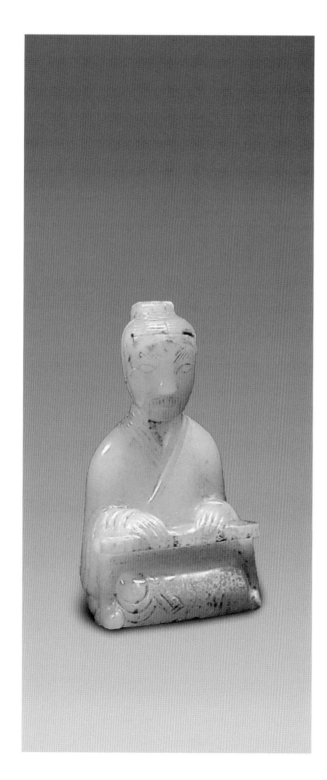

坐形白玉人

西汉

玉质

高 5.4 厘米

White Jade Seated Figurine

Western Han Dynasty

Jade

Height 5.4 cm

通体由白玉制成。玉人脸型清瘦，长眉短须。发束于脑后，头戴小冠，冠带扎于颌下。身穿右衽长衣，腰系方格纹带。凭几而坐，双手置于几上。底座下阴刻铭文五行十字："维古玉人王公延十九年"。

河北博物院藏

The figurine is made of white jade. The figurine with a thin face, long eyebrows and short beard wears a little crown whose ply is tied under the jaw, long suits in right overlapping part, and a checkered pattern belt. He is sitting by a tea table with his hands on it. The base is inscribed with ten Chinese characters "Wei Gu Yu Ren Wang Gong Yan Shi Jiu Nian" describing the figurine.

Preserved in Hebei Museum

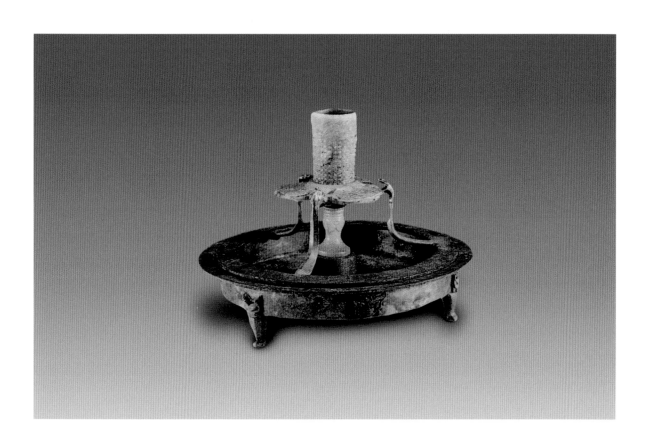

承露玉杯

西汉

铜质、金银质、玉质

通高 17 厘米

Jade Dew-gathering Cup

Western Han Dynasty

Bronze, gold, silver and jade

Height 17 cm

由青铜圆盘、银嵌金兽形架和高足玉杯组成。
青铜圆盘直口，宽折沿，平底，下有三兽形足。
银嵌金兽形架接于盘上，呈三条张口蛇的形
象。玉杯呈黄色，置于盘中，以架固定，直口，
深腹，高足，杯壁上饰乳钉纹。此杯是承接
露水供帝王饮用的器具。

西汉南越王博物馆藏

The collection consists of a bronze disc, a gold
beast-shaped frame inlaid with silver, and a
jade stem cup. The bronze disc has a straight
mouth, a wide and flat rim, a flat bottom, and
three animal-shaped feet. The gold beast-shaped
frame inlaid with silver rests on the pan with
three mouth-opening snakes. The yellow jade
cup, which is placed on a tray, has a straight
mouth, a deep belly, a high foot, and a wall
decorated with nail designs. The collection
was an appliance used for gathering dew for
imperial consumption.

Preserved in Museum of the Western Han Dynasty
Mausoleum of the Nanyue King

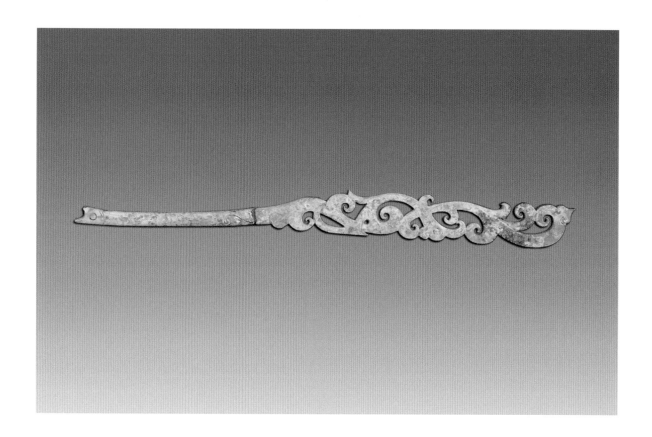

白玉镂空云凤纹笄

西汉

玉质

残长 19.2 厘米，宽 1.6 厘米，厚 0.5 厘米

White Jade Hollow Hairpin Patterned with Phoenix and Clouds

Western Han Dynasty

Jade

Residual Length 19.2 cm/ Width 1.6 cm/ Thickness 0.5 cm

通体由白玉制成，光洁无瑕。首部透雕凤鸟卷云纹，上涂有朱砂痕迹，有圆孔，已残。器物玲珑剔透，线条流畅。用以绾定发髻或冠。

河北博物院藏

The bright and flawless hairpin is made of white jade. The head is carved with patterns of phoenix and cirrus clouds, on which is coated with cinnabar. Had a hole on it, the hairpin is slightly damaged. This exquisitely carved hairpin with smooth lines was used for fixing bun or crown.

Preserved in Hebei Museum

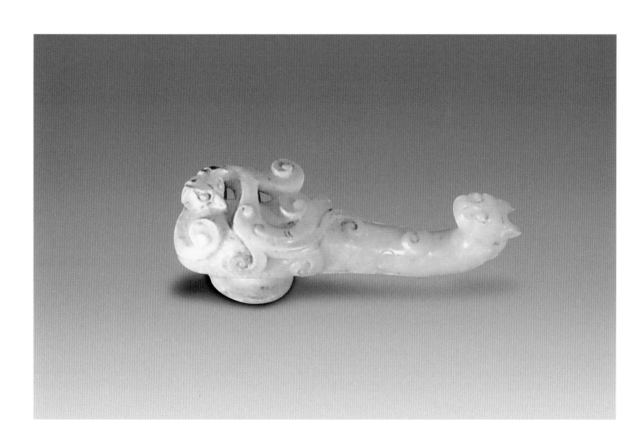

白玉兽纹带钩

西汉

玉质

长 5.8 厘米，厚 1.8 厘米

White Jade Belt Hook with Animal Patterns

Western Han Dynasty

Jade

Length 5.8 cm/ Thickness 1.8 cm

通体白玉制成，细腻莹润。钩首琢呈兽首形，钩背高浮雕一只朱雀。两侧阴刻卷云纹，表面有朱砂痕迹。

河北博物院藏

This fine and moisturized hook is made of white jade. The head and the back of the hook are carved with an animal's head and a scarlet bird in high relief. Cirrus clouds are incised on both sides, on the surface of which there are cinnabar marks.

Preserved in Hebei Museum

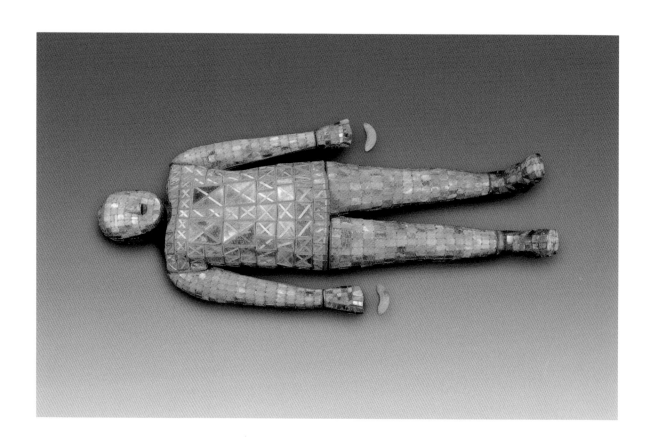

窦绾金缕玉衣

西汉

玉质

全长 172 厘米

Dou Wan's Jade Clothes Sewn with Gold Thread

Western Han Dynasty

Jade

Length 172 cm

为中山靖王刘胜妻窦绾下葬时所穿的金缕玉
衣。玉片为岫岩玉，多数呈纯绿色，夹有灰白、
黄褐色。玉衣分为五部分。共用玉片 2160 片，
金丝约 700 克。玉衣形式与刘胜墓的相似，
头下有鎏金镶玉铜枕。1968 年河北省满城陵
山中山靖王刘胜妻窦绾墓出土。

河北博物院藏

The jade clothes were worn by Dou Wan, the
wife of Liu Sheng (the King of Zhongshan),
when she was buried. The slices are made of
Xiuyan jade and are mostly pure green dotted
with gray or brown. The jade clothes consist of
five parts with a total of 2,160 jade slices and 700-
gram gold thread. The style of the jade clothes
is similar to that of the clothes in Liu Sheng's
Tomb. There is a gilt bronze pillow inlaid with
jade under the head. The artifact was excavated
from Dou Wan's Tomb in Mount Ling, Mancheng
District, Hebei Province, in 1968.

Preserved in Hebei Museum

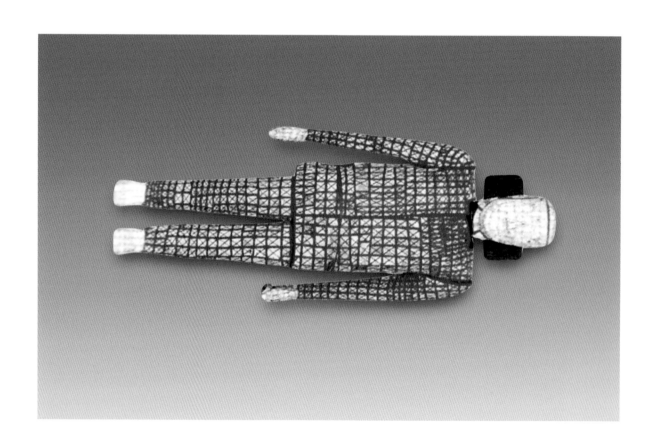

丝缕玉衣

西汉

玉质

通长 173 厘米，肩宽 44 厘米

Jade Clothes Sewn with Silk Thread

Western Han Dynasty

Jade

Length 173 cm/ Shoulder Width 44 cm

为南越王赵眜下葬时所穿玉衣。由头套、衣身、手套、袖筒、裤筒和鞋等多部组合为一，计用玉片 2291 块，以丝线通过玉片上的穿孔编缕而成。1983 年广州象山岗南越王赵眜墓出土。

西汉南越王博物馆藏

The Nanyue King Zhao Mo wore the jade clothes when he was buried. The clothes are a combination of cap, suit, gloves, sleeves, legs of pants, shoes and other parts. The 2,291 jade slices were threaded with silk through their perforations. The artifact was excavated from the tomb of the Nanyue King Zhao Mo in Xiangshangang of Guangzhou City, Guangdong Province, in 1983.

Preserved in Museum of the Western Han Dynasty Mausoleum of the Nanyue King

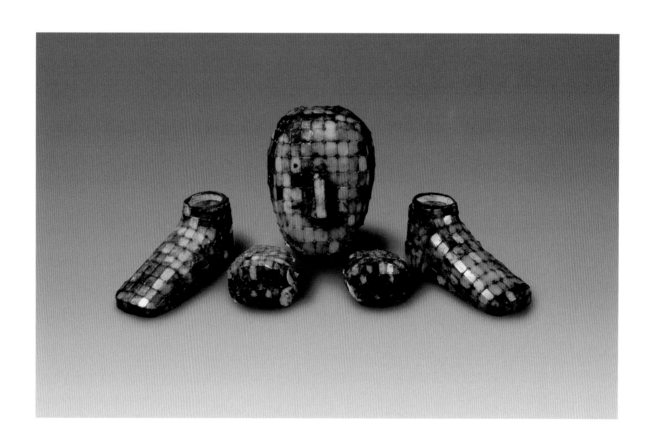

刘疵金缕玉罩

西汉

玉质

头罩高 27 厘米，足罩长 28 厘米，手罩长 14.5 厘米

Liu Ci's Jade Shields Sewn with Gold Thread

Western Han Dynasty

Jade

Hood Height 27 cm/ Shoe Length 28 cm/ Glove Length 14.5 cm

为刘疵下葬时所着玉罩，由头罩、足罩、手罩 5 件组成。1140 块玉片中，除头罩顶部用一块小玉璧外，均为三角形、方形和长方形的玉片用金缕编缀而成。玉片较薄，呈青色，表面光滑素雅。山东临沂刘疵墓出土，根据墓中出土刘疵玛瑙印可知墓主人。

临沂市博物馆藏

Liu Ci wore these jade shields when he was buried. They consist of five pieces: a hood, a pair of shoes, and a pair of gloves. The 1,140 jade slices are pieces of triangles, squares, and rectangles woven with gold thread, except for a small piece of jade on the hook. The thin and green jade slices have a smooth and plain surface. The collection was excavated from Liu Ci's Tomb in Linyi City, Shandong Province. The owner of the tomb can be identified based on Liu Ci's agate seal in the tomb.

Preserved in Linyi Museum

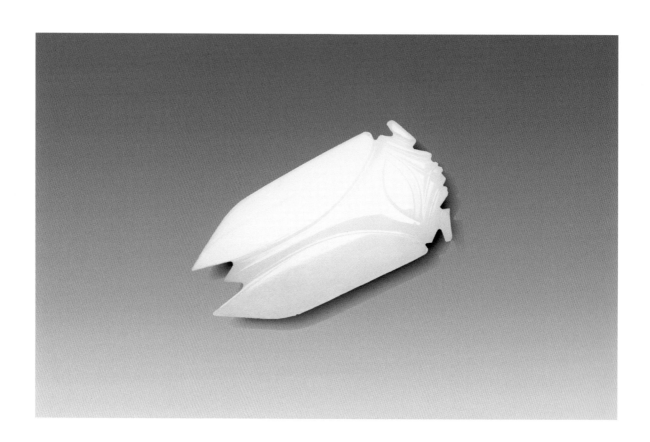

蝉形玉琀

西汉

玉质

长 5.7 厘米，宽 2.9 厘米

Cicada-shaped Jade Han

Western Han Dynasty

Jade

Length 5.7 cm/ Width 2.9 cm

琀呈蝉形，用新疆和田玉琢成，洁白无瑕，光质莹润，具有极强的透明感，蝉头部略呈弧形，眼目突出，嘴角分明，弧线形的蝉翼覆盖着蝉身。蝉腹部刻有十二道弧形内凹的横纹，表现出蝉的有伸缩功能的腹节。琀为古代的一种葬玉，通常呈蝉形，含在死者口中。古人认为玉是山川之精华，置于人的口中，使人的精气不会外泄，尸身不会腐烂，希望死后能像蝉那样高洁、蜕变，以求来世再生。1988 年出土于杭州市邗江县（今邗江区）甘泉乡姚庄西汉木椁墓。

扬州博物馆藏

The cicada-shaped Han, which is made of Xinjiang Hetian jade, is pure white, flawless and transparent. The cicada has a slightly curved head, protruding eyes and mouth, and arc wings. The cicada's abdomen is engraved with twelve concave stripes, showing the contractible abdominal segment of the cicada. Han, a cicada-shaped jade burial object in ancient time, was kept in the deceased's mouth. It is believed that placing jade, the essence of mountains, in a person's mouth can prevent the vital essence from releasing and the body from decaying. People wished that they would be noble like the metamorphosis of the cicada and prayed for afterlife. The artifact was excavated from a timber-chambered tomb of the Western Han Dynasty in Ganquan Village of Hanjiang County (now Hanjiang District), Yangzhou City, in 1988. Preserved in Yangzhou Museum

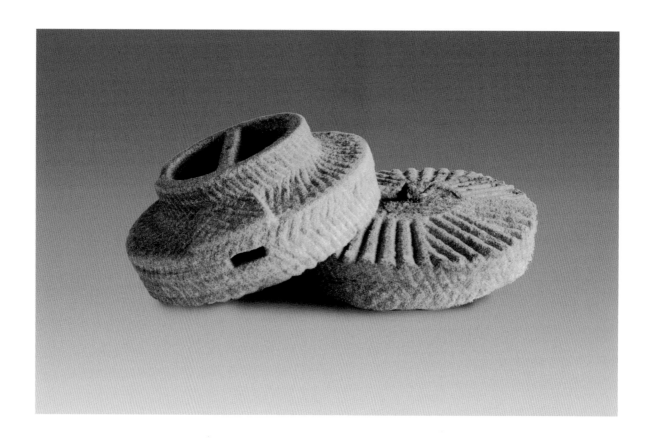

石磨

东汉

石质

直径 23 厘米，高 13.5 厘米

Stone Mill

Eastern Han Dynasty

Stone

Diameter 23 cm/ Height 13.5 cm

夹砂麻石凿磨而成，分为上下两片，器形规整，结合面凿出凹槽以便加大摩擦力。此磨盘造型古朴，凿工精细，结构合理，与近代石磨造型相差不大。为古代不可多见的日常生活用具。

李毓麟藏

The mill is made of sand granite by chiseling and grinding. It is regularly shaped and divided into two pieces whose joint surface is carved concave in order to increase friction. This mill has unadorned modeling, fine chiseling and proper structure. Its shape is similar to that of the modern mill. It was a valuable utensil of daily life in ancient time.

Collected by Li Yulin

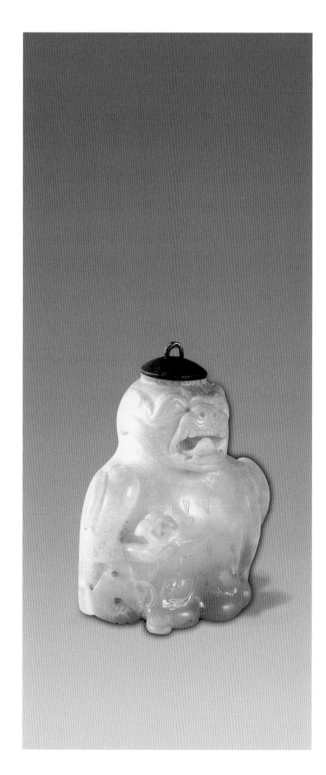

避邪形玉壶

东汉

玉质

长 6 厘米，宽 4.5 厘米，高 6.8 厘米，通高 7.7 厘米

Jade Pixie Pot

Eastern Han Dynasty

Jade

Length 6 cm/ Width 4.5 cm/ Height 6.8 cm/ Total

Height 7.7 cm

新疆和田白玉质。造型以一避邪呈跪坐状。右手托灵芝仙草，中部镂空，头顶开圆口，上置环钮，银盖。避邪身刻细圆圈纹、羽毛纹，集圆雕、镂空、浮雕、阴线细刻手法于一体。为东汉玉器的杰作。1984 年扬州市邗江区甘泉老虎墩东汉墓出土。

扬州博物馆藏

The pot, which is made of Xinjiang Hetian jade, is shaped like a bixie a winged lion-like beast, kneeling with its right hand holding lucid ganoderma and fairy grass. Its middle part is hollowed out, and on the top of its head there is a round opening with a silver lid and a ring-shaped knob. The beast is carved with thin circle patterns and feather patterns, which combine such techniques as circular engravure, hollowing, carved relief and fine carving in shade line all in one. As a jade masterpiece of the Eastern Han Dynasty, the pot was excavated from Ganquan Laohudun Tomb of the Eastern Han Dynasty, Hanjiang District of Yangzhou City, in 1984.

Preserved in Yangzhou Museum

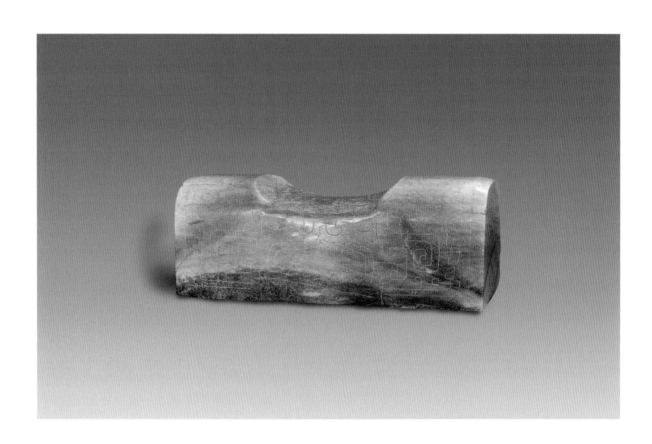

青玉云纹枕

东汉

玉质

长 34.7 厘米，宽 11.8 厘米，高 13 厘米，重 13800 克

Cyan Jade Pillow with Cloud Pattern

Eastern Han Dynasty

Jade

Length 34.7 cm/ Width 11.8 cm/ Height 13 cm/ Weight 13,800 g

器用整块青玉雕制而成。枕中部内凹，枕面
及前、后两面均以细而浅的双勾阴线刻出宛
转流畅、相互勾连的变形云纹。

河北博物院藏

The pillow was carved out of a whole piece
of cyan jade. In the front, at the back, and on
both sides of the pillow with a dented center
are smooth interlocked cloud patterns engraved
with fine and shallow double hook lines.

Preserved in Hebei Museum

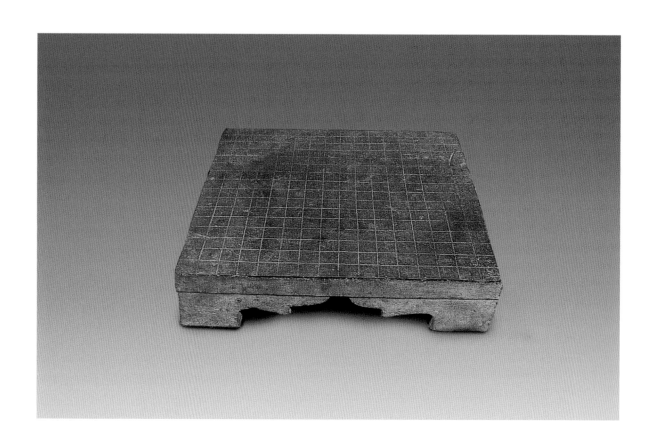

石围棋盘

东汉

石质

宽 69 厘米，高 14 厘米

Stone Board of Go

Eastern Han Dynasty

Stone

Width 69 cm/ Height 14 cm

棋盘为石质。盘面呈正方形，上有纵、横各十七道的经纬线组成盘局，盘下有四足。这是目前考古发现中时代较早的围棋盘实物。1952 年河北省望都县东汉墓出土。

望都汉墓博物馆藏

This stone board of go has a square surface that consists of 17 horizontal lines and 17 vertical lines. The board is supported by four feet. This is a relatively early material object of go board among the archaeological discoveries by far. The board was excavated from a tomb of the Eastern Han Dynasty in Wangdu County, Hebei Province, in 1952.

Preserved in Wangdu Museum of Han Dynasty Mausoleum

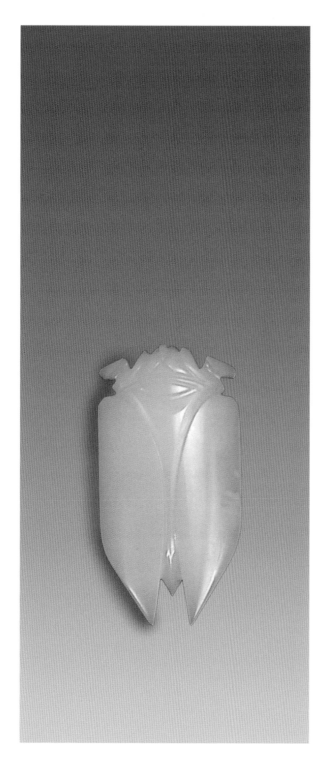

蝉形玉琀

东汉

玉质

长 6.4 厘米，宽 3.3 厘米

Cicada-shaped Jade Han

Eastern Han Dynasty

Jade

Length 6.4 cm/ Width 3.3 cm

琀呈蝉形，用新疆和田玉琢成，洁白无瑕，晶莹剔透，具有极强的透明感。用斜磨阴刻线条勾出头、胸、腹、双翼等细部轮廓。蝉头部略呈弧形，双目外凸，嘴角分明，弧线形的蝉翼覆盖着蝉身。蝉腹部刻有十二道弧形内凹的横纹，表现出蝉的有伸缩功能的腹节。蝉尾和翼端呈尖锋状。

河北博物院藏

The cicada-shaped Han, which is made of Xinjiang Hetian jade, is pure white, flawless and very transparent. The cicada's head, chest, abdomen, and wings were carved with incised lines. The cicada has a slightly curved head, protruding eyes and mouth, and arc wings. Its abdomen is engraved with twelve concave stripes, showing the contractible abdominal segment of the cicada. The cicada has spike-shaped wings and a tail end.
Preserved in Hebei Museum

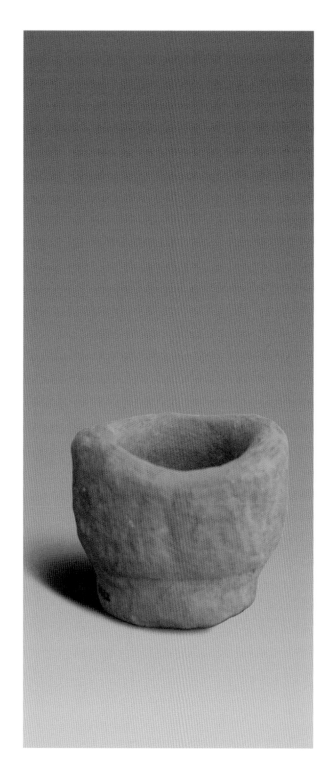

石臼

汉

石质

口径 18 厘米，底径 14 厘米，通高 16 厘米，重 1110 克

Stone Mortar

Han Dynasty

Stone

Mouth Diameter 18 cm/ Bottom Diameter 14 cm/

Height 16 cm/ Weight 1,110 g

通体敲琢而成，未经磨制。直口，直腹，平底。
为生活器具。陕西省澄城县征集。

陕西医史博物馆藏

The mortar was carved without grinding. As a household appliance, it has a straight mouth, a straight belly, and a flat bottom. The mortar was collected in Chengcheng County, Shaanxi Province.

Preserved in Shaanxi Museum of Medical History

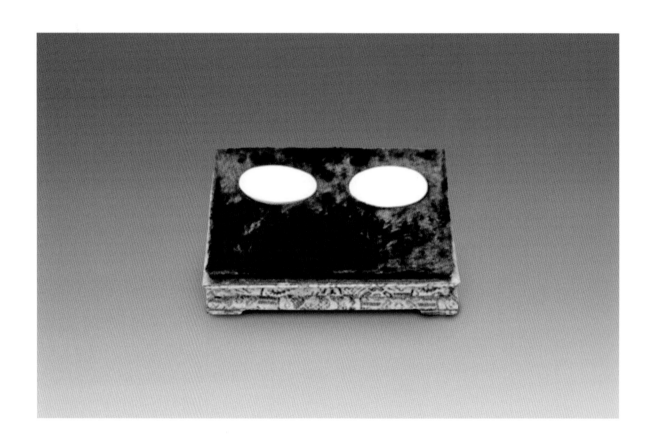

玉眼罩

汉

玉质

长径 4.4 厘米，短径 2.4 厘米

Jade Eye Patches

Han Dynasty

Jade

Long Diameter 4.4 cm/ Short Diameter 2.4 cm

眼罩一对，形制完全一致，由白玉磨制而成，椭圆形，光滑规整。我国古人以玉为天地之精英，常有吞食玉屑以期长生者，并有死后佩于遗体者。周时有以玉器掩闭尸体之眼、耳、口、鼻及前后二阴，谓可以防止死后腐液之外流，此即掩于尸眼之玉罩，其传世约历三千年。

广东中医药博物馆藏

This pair of smooth and regular eye patches are of exactly the same oval shape. It is made of white jade. Ancient Chinese people believed that jade was the essence of the universe. Therefore, people often swallowed jade chips to pray for a long life and wore jade objects after death. In the Zhou Dynasty, jade was used to cover eyes, ears, nose, mouth, and the urethral and anal orifices of dead body in order to prevent rotten liquid from draining from the body after death. The cadaver-covering jade patches were conserved for at least 3,000 years.

Preserved in Guangdong Chinese Medicine Museum

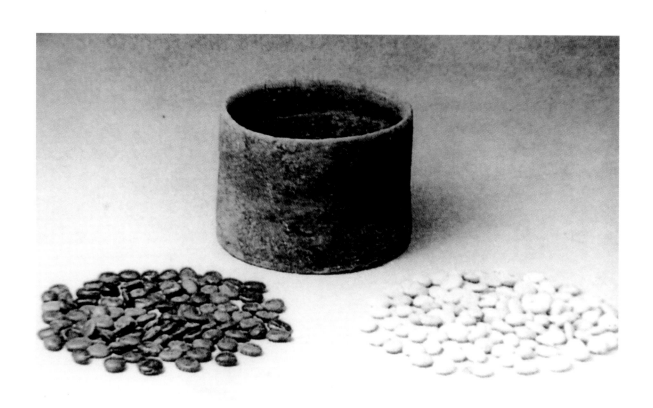

石围棋子

西晋

石质

直径约 1 厘米，厚约 0.2 厘米

Stone Pieces of Go

Western Jin Dynasty

Stone

Diameter about 1 cm/ Thickness about 0.2 cm

用黑、白石子磨制而成。扁圆形，共
二百七十二枚，表面光滑圆润，出土时装于
灰陶罐内。罐为直口，深腹，平底。这套围
棋子是中国较早的围棋实物。1974 年山东省
邹县西晋永康二年（301）刘宝墓出土。

邹城市文物局藏

The stone pieces of go are made of black and
white pebbles by grinding. They add up to 272,
and are oblate, smooth and moisturized. They
are in a gray clay pot with a straight mouth, a
deep belly and a flat bottom. This set was earlier
material objects of go pieces in China. The
collection was excavated from Liu Bao's tomb of
the second year of Yongkang Period (301) of the
Western Jin Dynasty in Zou County, Shandong
Province, in 1974.

Preserved in Zoucheng Municipal Bureau of
Cultural Relics

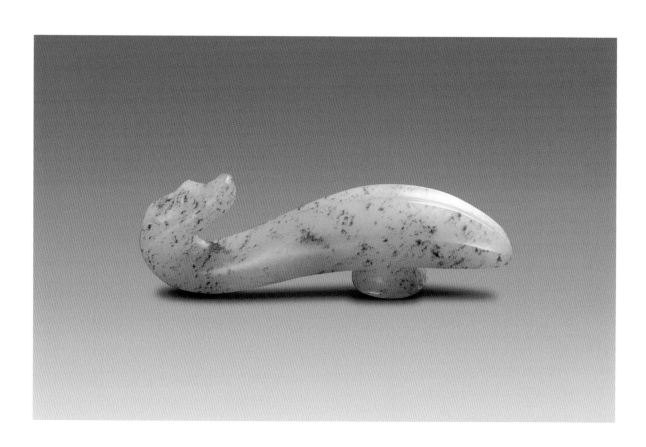

玉带钩

东晋

玉质

长 5.9 厘米，宽 1.6 厘米，高 1.9 厘米

Jade Belt Hook

Eastern Jin Dynasty

Jade

Length 5.9 cm/ Width 1.6 cm/ Height 1.9 cm

玉质白色温润，半透明，间有土沁褐斑。钩
首呈兽首回顾状，钩体饰简化羽翼。东晋侍
中高崧墓出土，是该墓所出遗物中质地最佳
的玉器之一。

南京市博物馆藏

The jade with brown spots is white, mellow,
and semi-translucent. The head of the hook
is that of a beast which is turning back. The
body of the hook is decorated with simplified
wings. The hook was excavated from the tomb
of Gao Song, privy counselor in the Eastern Jin
Dynasty. It is one of the best jades unearthed in
this tomb.

Preserved in Nanjing Municipal Museum

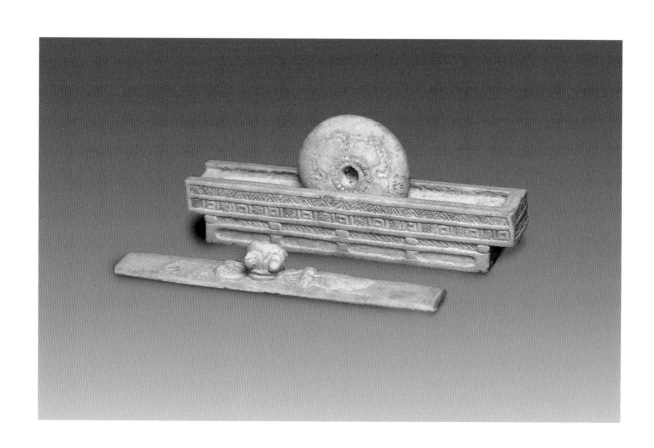

药碾

唐

玉质

碾：长 26.5 厘米，宽 5.5 厘米，高 8 厘米

轮：直径 9 厘米，槽深 2 厘米，孔直径 1 厘米

Medicine Roller

Tang Dynasty

Jade

Roller: Length 26.5 cm/ Width 5.5 cm/ Height 8 cm

Wheel: Diameter 9 cm/ Depth of the Groove 2 cm/

Diameter of the Roller Hole 1 cm

整体由汉白玉雕成，由碾身、碾盖和碾轮组成。碾身呈方形，表面饰云雷纹。碾盖为插入型。碾轮中部有圆孔，使用时可在圆孔中插入圆棒。1984 年河北省晋县（今晋州市）唐墓出土。

晋州市文物局藏

The collection, which was carved out of Han white jade, consists of the body, a cover and a wheel. The square body of the roller has a surface with thunder cloud patterns. The cover is of plug-in type. In the middle of the wheel there is a round hole, into which a round rod could be inserted when in use. The collection was excavated from a tomb of the Tang Dynasty in Jin County (now Jinzhou City), Hebei Province, in 1984.

Preserved in Jinzhou Municipal Bureau of Cultural Relics

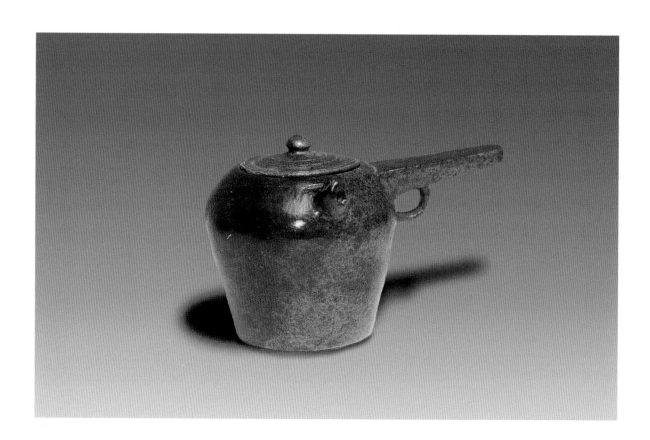

煎药壶

唐

石质

口径 8.5 厘米，腹径 13.5 厘米，底径 10.5 厘米，高 14.8 厘米，腹深 12 厘米，把长 11 厘米

Medicine-decocting Pot

Tang Dynasty

Stone

Mouth Diameter 8.5 cm/ Belly Diameter 13.5 cm/ Bottom Diameter 10.5 cm/ Height 14.8 cm/ Belly Depth 12 cm/ Handle Length 11 cm

由一块完整石材雕琢、磨制而成。腹上端有一个壶嘴，药水可倒出。手柄与壶身联结处的下端有一个石环起连接和支撑作用。

首都博物馆藏

The pot was carved out of a whole rock. There is a spout on the upper part of the belly, from which medicinal water could be poured out. At the bottom of the joint of the handle and the body, there is a stone ring that serves to connect and support.

Preserved in The Capital Museum

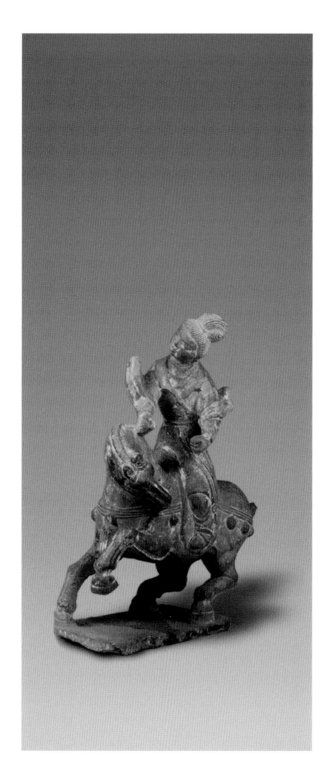

石雕女竞马俑

唐

石质

高 32.2 厘米

Stone Female Figurine in Horse Racing

Tang Dynasty

Stone

Height 32.2 cm

由一整块黄色石料雕琢而成，表现女骑手昂首用力勒马之情景。女骑手头梳高髻，面带微笑，低头俯视，内着紧袖衫，外穿开领交衽宽袖长裙。胯下奔马，背覆鞍具，呈竞驰中骤停状。造型生动逼真，极具特色。山东省济南市出土。

济南市博物馆藏

This figurine, which was carved out of a whole yellow rock, shows that a female rider is drawing the rein with her head holding high. She is wearing a smile and looking down with her hair tied up. She is wearing a tightly-sleeved shirt inside and an intersecting lapel dress with the open neck and loose sleeves. The horse stops suddenly in the air with a saddle on the back. The characteristic figurine was depicted vividly and almost to real. It was excavated in Jinan City, Shandong Province.

Preserved in Jinan Museum

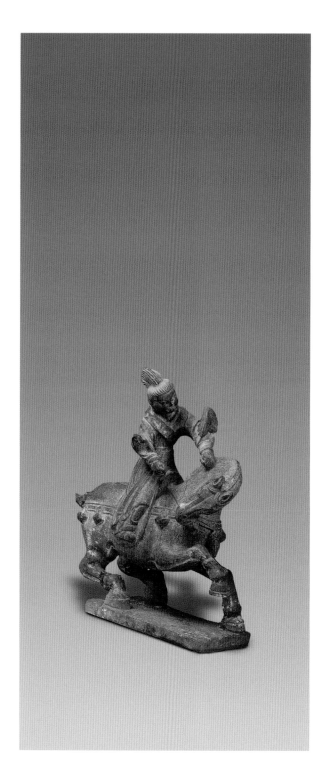

石雕女竞马俑

唐

石质

高 32.2 厘米

Stone Female Figurine in Horse Racing

Tang Dynasty

Stone

Height 32.2 cm

由一整块黄色石料雕琢而成，表现女骑手昂首用力勒马之情景。女骑手头梳高髻，面带微笑，低头俯视，内着紧袖衫，外穿开领交衽宽袖长裙。胯下奔马，背覆鞍具，呈竞驰中骤停状。造型生动逼真，极具特色。山东省济南市出土。

济南市博物馆藏

This figurine, which was carved out of a whole yellow rock, shows that a female rider is drawing the rein with her head holding up. She is wearing a smile and looking down with her hair tied up. She is wearing a tightly-sleeved shirt inside and an intersecting lapel dress with the open neck and loose sleeves. The horse stops suddenly in the air with a saddle on the back. The characteristic figurine was depicted vividly and almost to real. It was excavated in Jinan City, Shandong Province.

Preserve in Jinan Museum

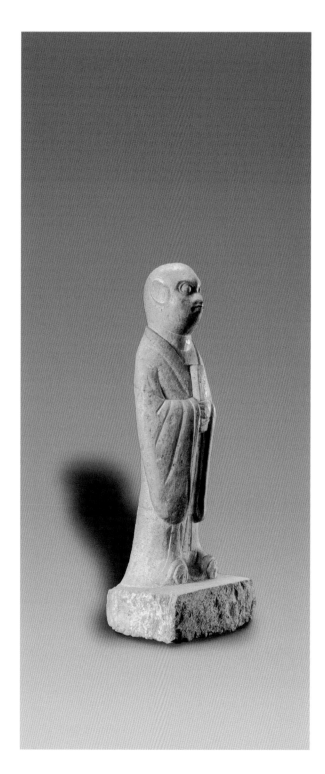

十二生肖之一——石刻猴像

唐

石质

高 42 厘米

Stone Monkey Statue

Tang Dynasty

Stone

Height 42 cm

猴，为十二生肖之一，是我国特有的民俗现
象之一。猴头，人身，身着对襟长袍，双手
执笏。

昭陵博物馆藏

The monkey is one of the 12 animal signs, a
unique Chinese fork custom. The statue has a
head like that of a monkey and a human body.
It wears a robe with buttons down the front and
holds a writing tablet in its hands.

Preserved in Zhao Tomb Museum

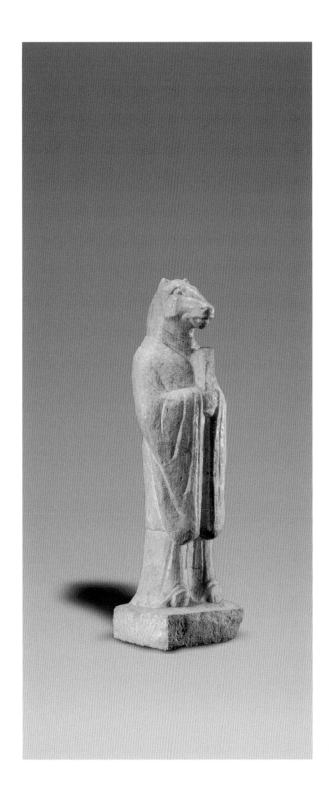

十二生肖之一——石刻马像

唐

石质

高 41 厘米

Stone Horse Statue

Tang Dynasty

Stone

Height 41 cm

马，为十二生肖之一，是我国特有的民俗现
象之一。马头，人身，身着对襟长袍，双手
执笏。

昭陵博物馆藏

The horse is one of the 12 animal signs, a unique
Chinese fork custom. The statue has a head like
that of a horse and a human body. It wears a
robe with buttons down the front and holds a
writing tablet in its hands.

Preserved in Zhao Tomb Museum

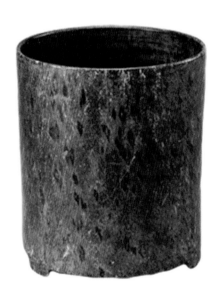

豹斑玉尊

北宋

玉质

直径 15.7 厘米，高 17.8 厘米

Jade Zun Patterned with Leopard Spots

Northern Song Dynasty

Jade

Diameter 15.7 cm/ Height 17.8 cm

黄褐色玉料制成，上有黑色杂质，形似豹斑。

圆筒状，直口，平底，下有方形短足。

武功县文物旅游局藏

The collection, made of brown jade material, has black impurities that resemble a leopard's spots. It is cylindrical, with a vertical mouth, a flat bottom, and square and short feet.

Preserved in Wugong County Cultural Relics and Tourism Bureau

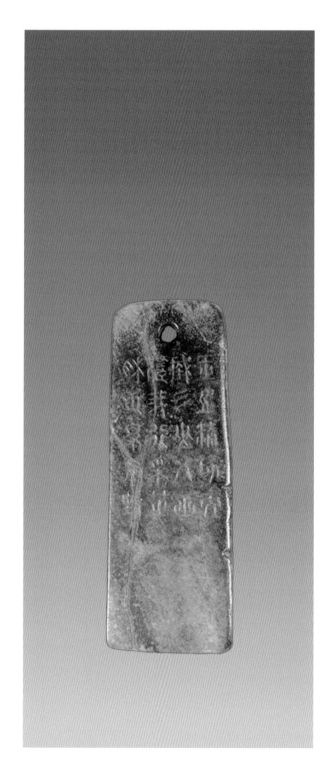

采芝玉铲

宋

玉质

长 15.8 厘米，宽 5.7 厘米，厚 0.8 厘米，圆孔
径 1 厘米

Jade Shovel for Collecting Ganoderma

Song Dynasty

Jade

Length 15.8 cm/ Width 5.7 cm/ Thickness 0.8 cm/

Hole Diameter 1 cm

以褐色玉料制成，近梯形，铲端有一圆孔，下部横削便于铲土。铲体刻有篆文："玉之精，琢而成，三山五岳随我行，采芝采卉得长生。"

上海中医药博物馆藏

The shovel, made of brown jade material, is almost ladder-shaped. There is a round hole at the top of it and the almost transverse peeling in the lower part makes it easy to shovel dirt. The shovel is engraved in seal script with words about the benefit of collecting ganoderma.

Preserved in Shanghai Museum of Traditional Chinese Medicine

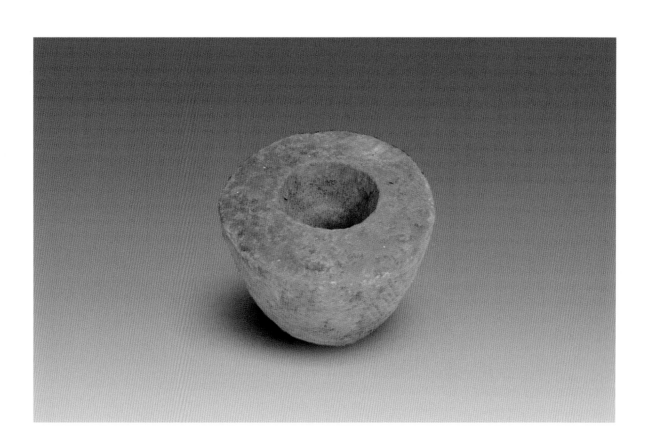

药臼

宋

石质

口径 23 厘米，高 16.5 厘米

Medicine Mortar

Song Dynasty

Stone

Mouth Diameter 23 cm/ Height 16.5 cm

由整块石材中挖空一块作为臼窝，敞口，平底，壁很厚。用于舂制药材。剑阁县文物管理所调拨。

成都中医药大学中医药传统文化博物馆藏

The mortar was hollowed out of the center of a stone. It has a flared mouth, a flat bottom, and a thick wall. The main function of the mortar was to pound medicinal herbs. It was allocated from Jiange County Office of Cultural Relics Preservation.

Preserved in Museum of Traditional Chinese Medicine Culture, Chengdu University of Traditional Chinese Medicine

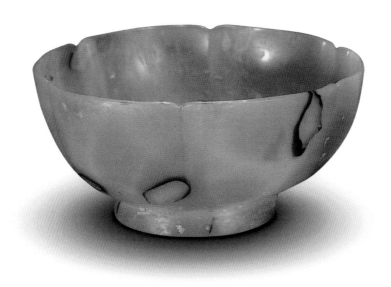

玛瑙花式碗

宋

玉质

口径 11.3 厘米，底径 5.7 厘米，通高 5 厘米

Agate Bowl with Flower Patterns

Song Dynasty

Jade

Mouth Diameter 11.3 cm/ Bottom Diameter 5.7 cm/ Height 5 cm

白色玛瑙制成，敞口，六瓣海棠花形，深腹，

圈足，内外壁均有紫红色的斑纹。质地致密，

晶莹剔透，造型典雅秀丽。

河北博物院藏

The bowl, which is made of white agate, has a deep belly and a ring foot. The everted mouth is like a begonia with six petals. The interior and exterior walls of the bowl have purple red streaks. The bowl has dense texture, a crystal clear body, and elegant modeling.

Preserved in Hebei Museum

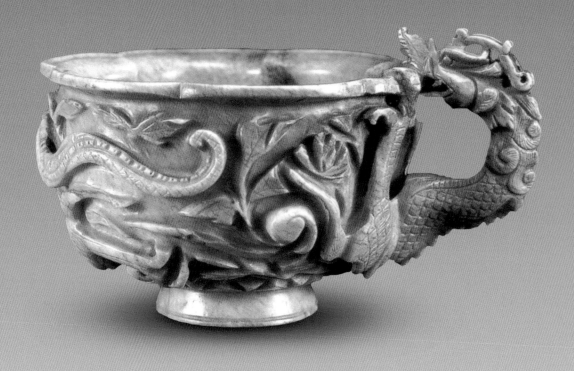

玉螭耳杯

宋

玉质

口径 9.5 厘米，高 6 厘米

由整块黄色玉料雕琢而成。直口，宽折沿，深腹，圈足。杯耳呈螭首状，螭身盘绕于杯腹，其间装饰以花卉纹。玉杯从唐代开始大量使用，此后各代形制基本沿袭前代，唯制作日趋精湛而已。由于文化观念的原因，宋代玉器少见螭这种非写实性题材，而以写实花卉装饰杯体居多。

故宫博物院藏

Jade Ear Cup with a Chi Dragon-patterned

Song Dynasty

Jade

Mouth Diameter 9.5 cm/ Height 6 cm

This cup, carved out of yellow jade material, has a straight mouth, a wide rhombic folded rim, a deep belly, and a ring foot. The ear of the cup is like the head of a Chi dragon and the dragon's body twines around the belly decorated with flower patterns. Jade cups began to be used in large quantities in the Tang Dynasty. In the subsequent dynasties, the basic shape followed that of the previous dynasty, but the production process became increasingly exquisite. Due to the cultural values, the non-realistic theme of legendary dragon was very rare in the Song Dynasty while realistic flowers always decorated the body of jade cups.

Preserved in The Palace Museum

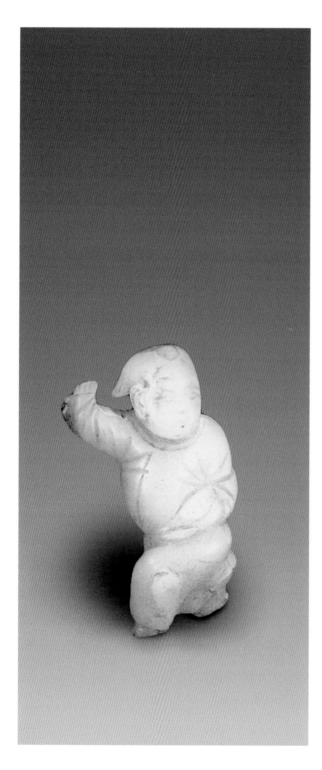

玉习武童子

宋

玉质

宽 3 厘米，高 5.7 厘米

Jade Boy Figurine Practicing Kung Fu

Song Dynasty

Jade

Width 3 cm/ Height 5.7 cm

童子为白玉雕成。短脸，后脑较大，身着肥大的衣裤。左腿下蹲，右掌推出，呈习练拳术形象。

故宫博物院藏

The boy figurine in sloppy clothes, made of white jade, has a short face and a larger afterbrain. Bending his left leg and pushing his right palm, he is making the posture of practicing kung fu.

Preserved in The Palace Museum

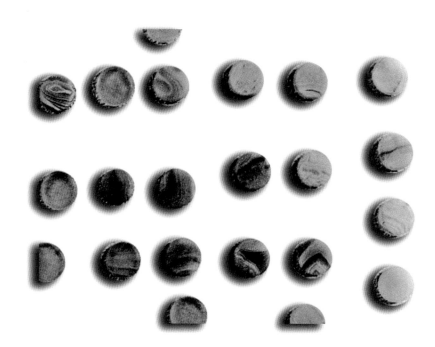

玛瑙围棋子

元

玉质

直径 1.45～1.8 厘米，厚 0.32～0.35 厘米

Agate Pieces of Go

Yuan Dynasty

Jade

Diameter 1.45–1.8 cm/ Thickness 0.32–0.35 cm

共出土围棋子 222 颗，皆两面扁平，其中红色
棋子 121 颗，为红玛瑙磨制而成；白色棋子
101 颗，为白玛瑙磨制。从出土地点来看，应
为封建统治阶级中上层人物所用之物。1972 年
北京后英房胡同元代居住遗址出土。

北京市文物研究所藏

The collection consists of 222 flat pieces of go.
There are 121 red pieces made of red agate and
101 white ones made of white agate. Judging from
the site of excavation, these pieces of go were used
by people of middle and upper ruling classes in
the feudal society. The collection was excavated
at Houyingfang alley residential site of the Yuan
Dynasty, Beijing, in 1972.
Preserved in Beijing Municipal Institute of
Cultural Relics

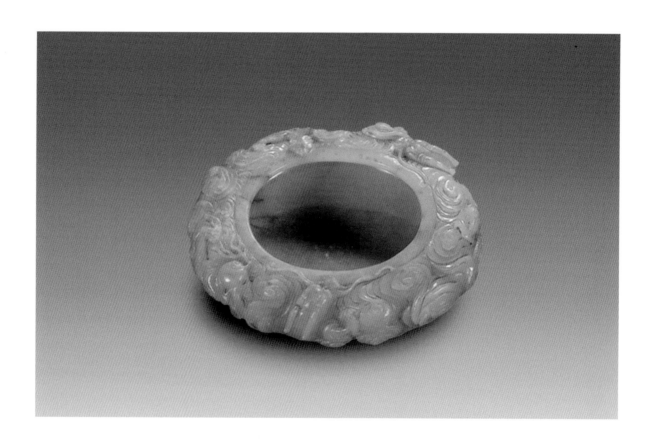

白玉雕龙洗

元

玉质

口径 9.3 厘米，腹径 16.5 厘米，高 4 厘米

White Jade Writing-brush Washer Patterned with Dragons

Yuan Dynasty

Jade

Mouth Diameter 9.3 cm/ Belly Diameter 16.5 cm/ Height 4 cm

以整块青白玉雕琢而成。椭圆形，敛口，鼓腹，平底。外壁雕琢二龙一螭，龙细部饰锯齿纹。

河北博物院藏

The washer was carved out of a green-white jade. It is oval with a contracted mouth, a bulged belly, and a flat bottom. The exterior wall was carved with two dragons and a Chi dragon decorated with sawtooth patterns.

Preserved in Hebei Museum

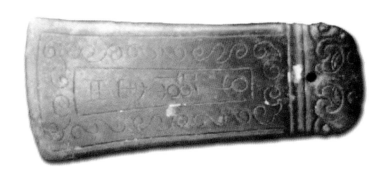

玉斧

明

玉质

长 10.4 厘米，最宽 4.5 厘米，厚 0.76 厘米，重 60 克

Jade Axe

Ming Dynasty

Jade

Length 10.4 cm/ Maximum Width 4.5 cm/ Thickness 0.76 cm/ Weight 60 g

青色玉料制成，斧身扁薄狭长，刃略呈弧形，两端上翘。斧首圆形，有穿孔。斧身刻有云纹，并刻有"子孙宝用""采药具"。

广东中医药博物馆藏

The axe, made of blue jade material, has a flat, thin and narrow body, an arc-shaped blade, and cocking-up ends. The round head of the axe is perforated and the body of axe is carved with cloud patterns and inscriptions "Zi Sun Bao Yong" (descendants' treasure) and "Cai Yao Ju" (tool for collecting medicinal herbs).

Preserved in Guangdong Chinese Medicine Museum

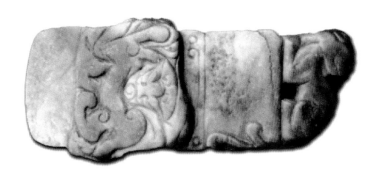

玉斧

明

玉质

长 11.36 厘米，宽 4.1 厘米，厚 1 厘米，重 125 克

Jade Axe

Ming Dynasty

Jade

Length 11.36 cm/ Width 4.1 cm/ Thickness 1 cm/ Weight 125 g

青色玉料制成。长方形，斧刃较短，中部及
一端刻有树叶、云纹饰。首端雕成一卧兽形。

广东中医药博物馆藏

The rectangular axe, which is made of blue jade
material, has a short blade. The center and one
end are carved with leaf and cloud patterns.
The head of the axe is carved with a crouching
beast.

Preserved in Guangdong Chinese Medicine Museum

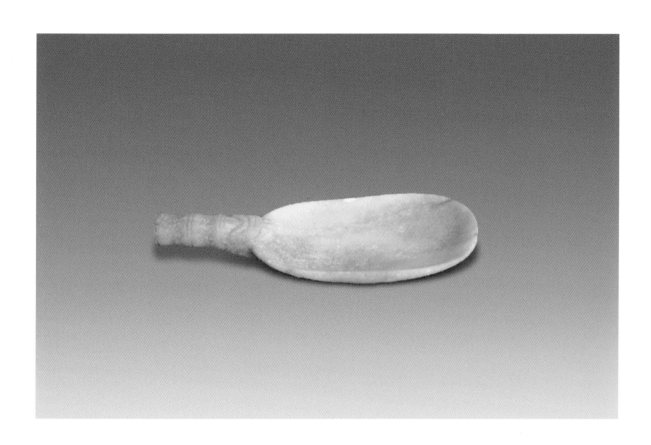

青玉药匙

明

玉质

长 15 厘米，深 2.5 厘米，重 118 克

Blue Jade Medicine Spoon

Ming Dynasty

Jade

Length 15 cm/ Depth 2.5 cm/ Weight 118 g

青玉药匙带底座，长方形药匙，圆角，有柄，柄呈竹节状。服药用。

广东中医药博物馆藏

The blue jade medicine spoon has a base and a round handle which is shaped like a bamboo with joints. The rectangular spoon was used for taking medicine.

Preserved in Guangdong Chinese Medicine Museum

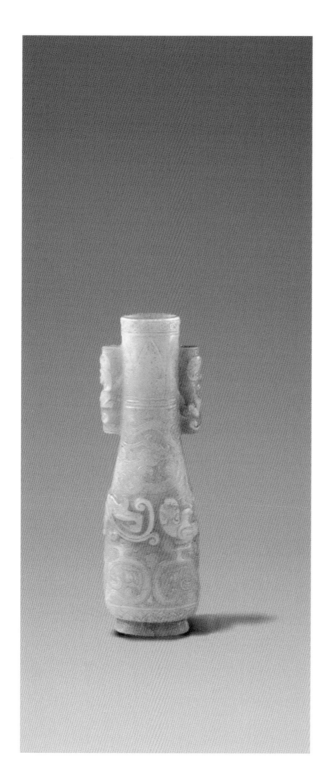

贯耳玉瓶

明

玉质

口径 3.1 ~ 3.7 厘米，高 18.7 厘米

Jade Bottle with Lugs on the Shoulders

Ming Dynasty

Jade

Mouth Diameter 3.1−3.7 cm/ Height 18.7 cm

青白玉雕琢而成。圆瓶，长颈，双贯耳，圈
足。通体饰纹，其中圈足、双耳雕螭龙纹，
瓶身刻双层浅浮雕，以龙纹、回纹、蕉叶纹、
仰莲纹为地纹，上浮雕螭龙纹。牛首山弘觉
寺塔地宫出土。

南京博物院藏

This round bottle, made of blue-white jade, has
a long neck, a pair of lugs on the shoulders,
and a ring foot. A hornless dragon patterns are
decorated on the ring foot and lugs. On the
body, there are two layers of bas-relief: dragon,
fret, banana-leaf, and lotus petal patterns in the
bottom and a hornless dragon patterns in bas-
relief at the top. The bottle was excavated from
the underground palace of Hongjue Pagoda in
Niushou Mountain, Nanjing City.

Preserved in Nanjing Museum

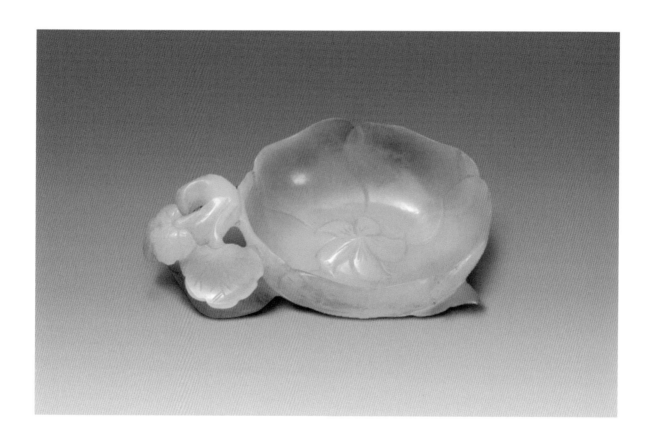

白玉花形杯

明

玉质

口径 7.3 厘米，高 3.2 厘米

White Jade Flower-shaped Cup

Ming Dynasty

Jade

Mouth Diameter 7.3 cm/ Height 3.2 cm

玉质晶莹，乳白色，洁净无瑕。杯呈盛开的
花朵，由 5 瓣相连，内底花蕊凸起，镂雕花
梗与叶梗为杯柄和杯托，柄上有数片嫩叶，
脉纹清晰。

山东博物馆藏

The jade is milky white and flawless. The
cup is shaped like a flower which has 5 petals
connected with each other. The protruding
stamens are on the bottom. The piercing
peduncle and leaf stalk are the handle and the
saucer of the cup, respectively. And on the
handle there are several tender leaves with clear
veins.

Preserved in Shandong Museum

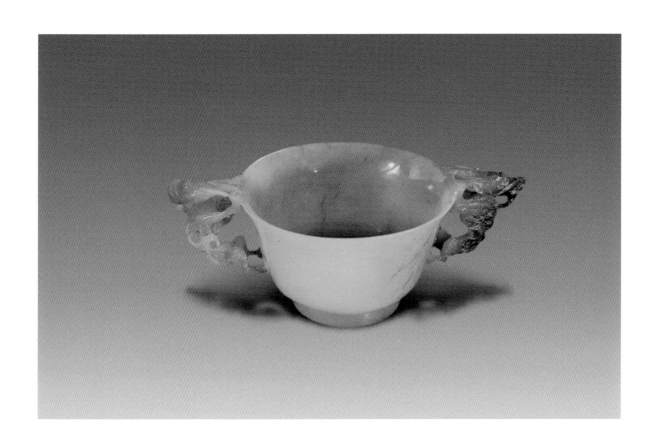

青玉双龙耳杯

明

玉质

口径 9.3 厘米，宽 15.1 厘米，高 5.2 厘米

Blue Jade Cup with Dragon-shaped Handles

Ming Dynasty

Jade

Mouth Diameter 9.3 cm/ Width 15.1 cm/ Height 5.2 cm

青玉雕琢而成，间有褐色。侈口，深腹，圈足，

左右双耳为透雕对称的双龙。

河北博物院藏

The cup is made of blue jade with a few brown
spots. The cup has a widely flared mouth, a deep
belly, a ring foot, and a pair of symmetrical
dragon-shaped handles.
Preserved in Hebei Museum

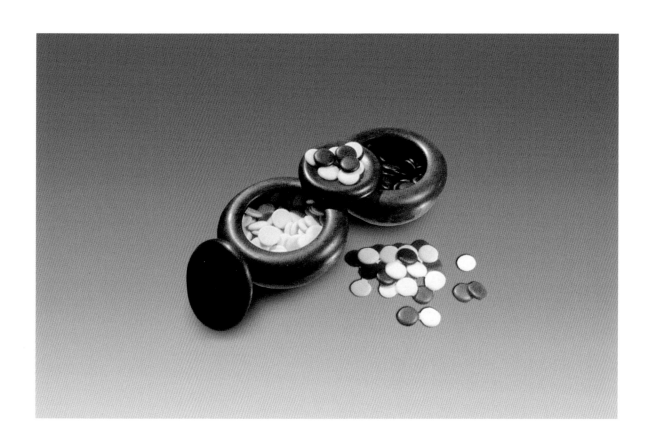

围棋

明

玉质

棋子：直径 2.2 厘米，厚 0.4 厘米

Pieces of Go

Ming Dynasty

Jade

Go Piece: Diameter 2.2 cm/ Thickness 0.4 cm

棋子以料石磨制，共 350 颗，皆两面扁平。其中白色 173 颗，黑色 177 颗，分盛在两个木制的黑色漆盒内。

中国体育博物馆藏

The pieces of go, which are made of dressed stone by grinding, add up to 350. Their two sides are flat. And there are 173 pieces in white and 177 in black, which are in two black wooden lacquered boxes separately.

Preserved in China Sports Museum

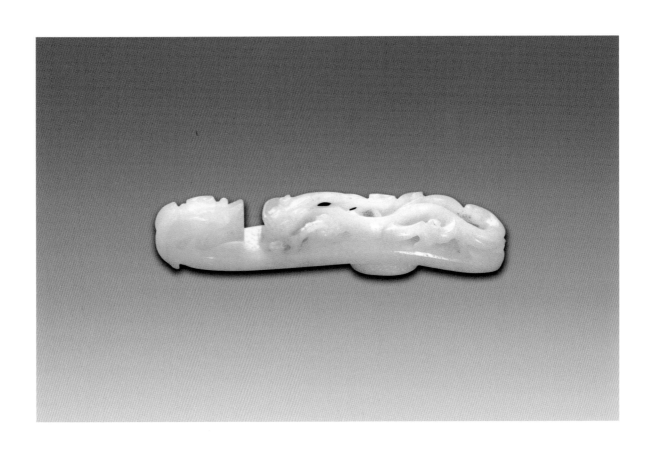

玉带钩

明

玉质

长 10 厘米

Jade Belt Hook

Ming Dynasty

Jade

Length 10 cm

白玉质，半透明状。带钩头部饰以龙首，龙角、
龙目突出，气势威严，线条刚劲利落。钩面
上饰蟠螭，体态盘曲伏卧，毛发上扬呈飘拂
状，四肢矫健有力。作品刀法细腻，形态优美。
南京市出土。

南京市博物馆藏

The white jade hook is translucent. Its head is
decorated with a dragon's head. The horn and
eyes of the dragon are protruding and majestic.
The lines are forceful and clear. The hook
surface is decorated with patterns of a hornless
dragon crouching tortuously. Its hair is blowing
in the air and its limbs are strong and powerful.
The style of cutting is fine and the dragon's
shape is graceful. The hook was excavated in
Nanjing.

Preserved in Nanjing Municipal Museum

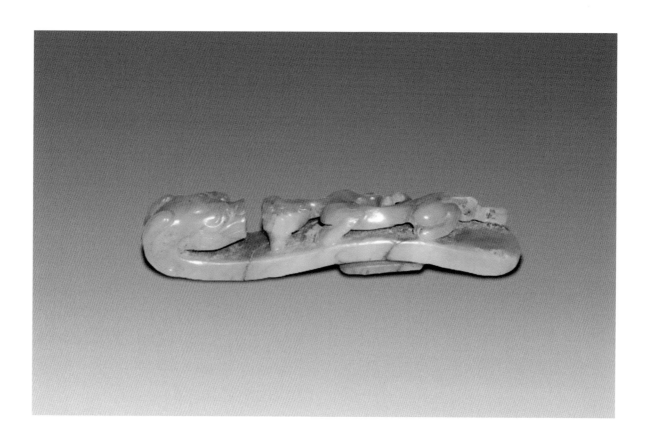

龙头螭纹玉带钩

明

玉质

长 11.1 厘米，宽 1.8～2.1 厘米，重 100 克

Jade Belt Hook with Patterns of the Head of Dragon and Chi

Ming Dynasty

Jade

Length 11.1 cm/ Width 1.8−2.1 cm/ Weight 100 g

白玉制成，呈"S"形。一端为兽头，面为
动物浮雕，背为蝉钮。有裂印。生活用器物。
1989 年入藏，级别为三级。陕西省咸阳市秦
都区公安局移交。

陕西医史博物馆藏

The S-shaped hook is made of white jade. One
end of it is a beast's head, the front surface of it
is animal relief, and the back surface is a cicada-
shaped button with cracks. The hook was used
in daily life. It was collected in the museum in
1989 and rated as Class 3. It was transferred by
the Public Security Bureau of Qindu District of
Xianyang City, Shaanxi Province.
Preserved in Shaanxi Museum of Medical History

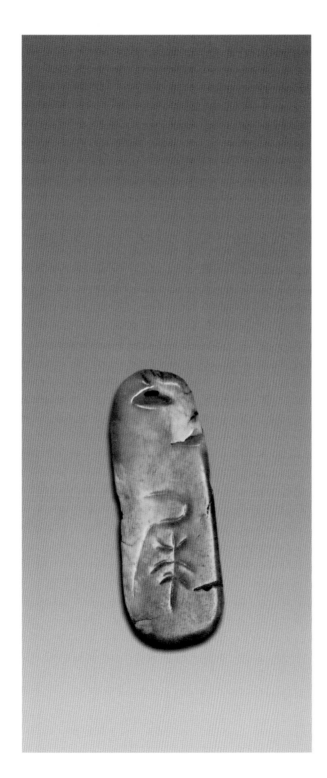

玉挂件

明

玉质

长 7.9 厘米，宽 3.55 厘米，厚 0.63 厘米

Jade Pendant

Ming Dynasty

Jade

Length 7.9 cm/ Width 3.55 cm/ Thickness 0.63 cm

黄色玉料制成。扁牌形，上刻一字，待考。
1960 年入藏。

　中华医学会 / 上海中医药大学医史博物馆藏

The pendant, which is made of yellow jade, is shaped like a plaque. There is a word (unverified) engraved on it. The pendant was collected by the museum in 1960.

Preserved in Chinese Medical Association/ Museum of Chinese Medicine, Shanghai University of Traditional Chinese Medicine

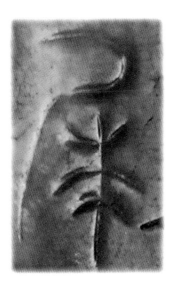

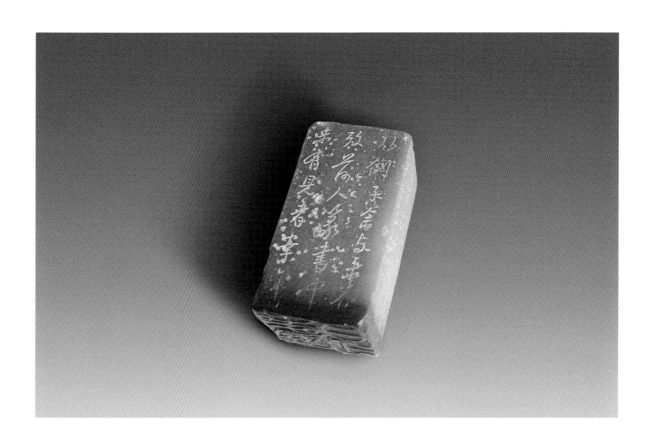

傅山刻"寒泉孤月"印章

明末清初

石质

长 3 厘米，宽 3 厘米，高 8 厘米

"Han Quan Gu Yue" Seal Carved by Fu Shan

Late Ming and Early Qing Dynasty

Stone

Length 3 cm/ Width 3 cm/ Height 8 cm

系明末清初医学家傅山所刻印章。黄色细
腻石料制成，整体为规整的长方体，侧面有
题词。

江苏省中医药博物馆藏

The seal was carved by the medical scientist Fu
Shan, who lived in the Late Ming and Early Qing
Dynasty. It is made of delicate yellow stone. The
whole body is a well-shaped rectangle, with
inscriptions on one lateral side.
Preserved in Jiangsu Museum of Traditional
Chinese Medicine

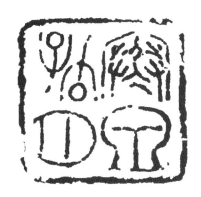

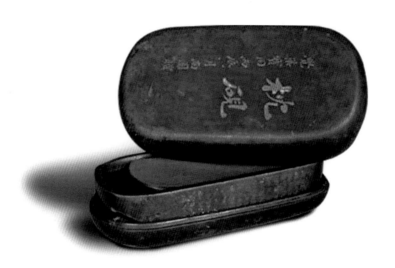

朱彝尊端石砚

清

石质

长 23.1 厘米，宽 14.4 厘米，厚 4 厘米

Zhu Yizun's Duanshi Inkstone

Qing Dynasty

Stone

Length 23.1 cm/ Width 14.4 cm/ Thickness 4 cm

该砚台为清代文学家、养生家朱彝尊之端石砚，黑色细腻石料制成，椭圆形。砚台外有红木盒套，盒盖刻有"枕砚""觉巢宝用丙辰八月南园赠"字样。朱彝尊（1629—1701），清文学家，秀水（今浙江嘉兴）人，少年时肆力古学，博览群书，康熙年间参与撰修《明史》，著有食疗书《食宪鸿秘》，另著《曝书亭集》等。1961 年入藏。

中华医学会 / 上海中医药大学医史博物馆藏

This inkstone was owned by Zhu Yizun, a writer and a health expert in the Qing Dynasty. It is made of delicate black stone. Outside the oval inkstone is a mahogany box set. The lid of the box is inscribed with some words. Zhu Yizun (1629−1701), a learned man who came from Xiushui (Jiaxing City, Zhejiang Province), participated in compiling books on the history of the Ming Dynasty in Kangxi Reign. He was the author of several books including the book on dietary therapy *Shi Xian Hong Mi* (A Collection of Recipes) and *Pu Shu Ting Ji* (A Collection of Poems). The inkstone was collected by the museum in 1961.

Preserved in Chinese Medical Association/ Museum of Chinese Medicine, Shanghai University of Traditional Chinese Medicine

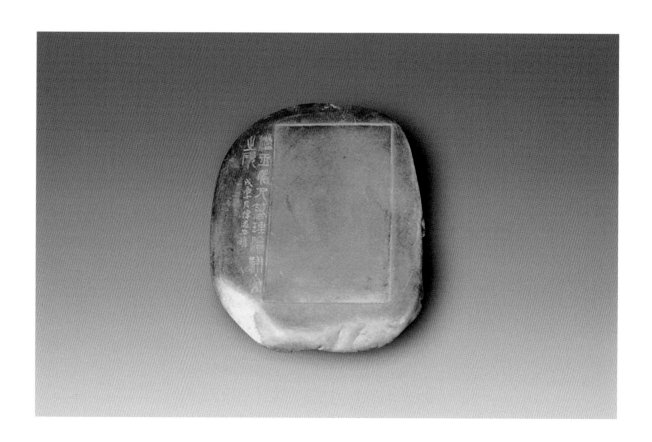

吴尚先用砚

清

石质

长 17 厘米，宽 12.5 厘米，高 2.5 厘米

Inkstone Used by Wu Shangxian

Qing Dynasty

Stone

Length 17 cm/ Width 12.5 cm/ Height 2.5 cm

此砚为清代医学家吴尚先著书时所用，为自然石块稍经加工制成，呈褐色，表面有光泽。背面左侧刻篆文 2 行 11 字："潜玉老人著理论骈文之砚"。左图为砚之拓片。

上海中医药博物馆藏

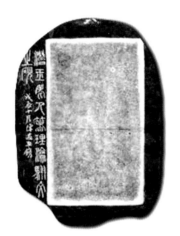

The brown inkstone was used by Wu Shangxian, a medical scientist in the Qing Dynasty, when he was writing books. It is made of natural stone by processing. It has a glossy surface and on the left side of its back are carved some words in seal script in two lines indicating the owner of the inkstone. The Left picture is the rubbing of the inkstone.

Preserved in Shanghai Museum of Traditional Chinese Medicine

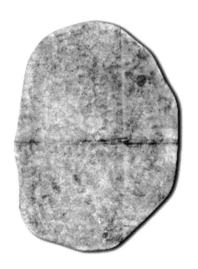

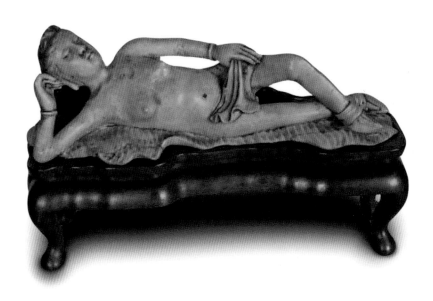

裸美

清

石质

长 24 厘米，宽 6 厘米

Stone of a Naked Woman

Qing Dynasty

Stone

Length 24 cm/ Width 6 cm

由整块黄色石料雕琢而成，表现为一个半侧卧的裸体妇女的形象。裸美是古代医生为妇女诊病时确定病痛部位的辅助工具。1956年入藏。

中华医学会／上海中医药大学医史博物馆藏

The collection, made of a whole yellow stone by grinding and chiseling, depicts the image of a naked woman lying on one side. The naked woman was used by the doctor as an auxiliary diagnostic tool to confirm where the pain was in the woman's body. The artifact was collected by the museum in 1956.

Preserved in Chinese Medical Association/ Museum of Chinese Medicine, Shanghai University of Traditional Chinese Medicine

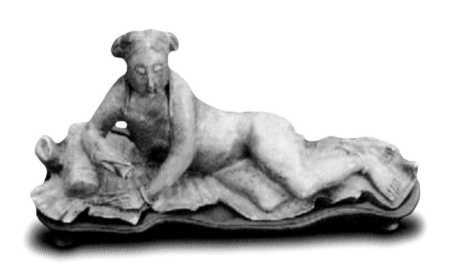

寿山石妇女像

清

石质

长 15.2 厘米，高 7.1 厘米，重 240 克

Shoushan Stone Woman Figurine

Qing Dynasty

Stone

Length 15.2 cm/ Height 7.1 cm/ Weight 240 g

由整块黄色石料雕琢而成，表现为一个半侧卧的半裸体妇女的形象。女子梳双髻，仅着肚兜，侧卧于席上。像下带底座。为摆件，装饰用。

广东中医药博物馆藏

The collection, which is made of a whole yellow stone by grinding and chiseling, depicts the image of a half-naked woman lying on one side. This woman with two hair knots is wearing a bellyband and lying on the mattress. The figurine has a base, which serves as decoration.

Preserved in Guangdong Chinese Medicine Museum

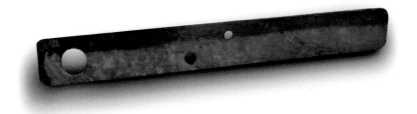

玉药铲

清

玉质

长 31.4 厘米，宽 3.95 厘米，厚 0.75 厘米

Jade Medicine Shovel

Qing Dynasty

Jade

Length 31.4 cm/ Width 3.95 cm/ Thickness 0.75 cm

该藏由整块墨绿色玉料制成，长板形。一端有
磨制刃口，另一端钻有一个大孔，中部钻有两
个小孔。通身磨制较好。1954 年入藏。

中华医学会 / 上海中医药大学医史博物馆藏

The collection is made of a whole dark green jade.
It is shaped like a long strip. There is a big hole on
one end of the shovel and a cutting edge on the other
end; two small holes are in the middle of the shovel.
It was collected in the museum in 1954.

Preserved in Chinese Medical Association/ Museum
of Chinese Medicine, Shanghai University of
Traditional Chinese Medicine

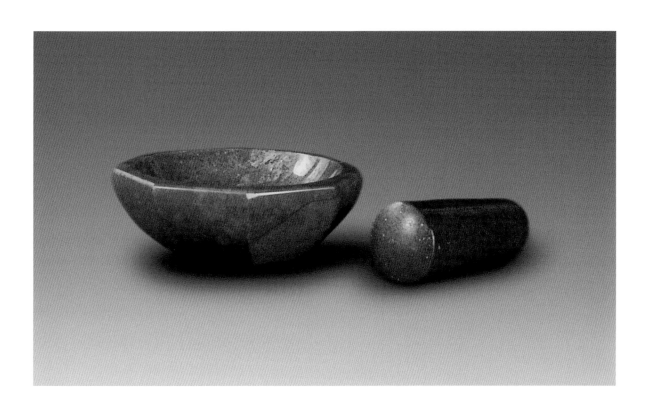

玛瑙研钵及杵

清

玉质

钵：口径 10 厘米，高 4.5 厘米

杵：长 7 厘米，最大直径 3.5 厘米

Agate Mortar and Pestle

Qing Dynasty

Jade

Mortar: Mouth Diameter 10 cm/ Height 4.5 cm

Pestle: Length 7 cm/ Maximum Diameter 3.5 cm

由质地坚硬的红色玛瑙制成。钵呈八边形，敞口，平底，壁较厚。杵呈圆棒状，一端大一端小。可用于研细一些较坚硬的药材。

上海中医药博物馆藏

The mortar and the pestle are made of hard red agate. The mortar is octagonal with a flared mouth, a flat bottom, and a thick wall. The pestle looks like a round stick with a big end and a small end. The mortar and the pestle were utilized for porphyrizing hard drug ingredients. Preserved in Shanghai Museum of Traditional Chinese Medicine

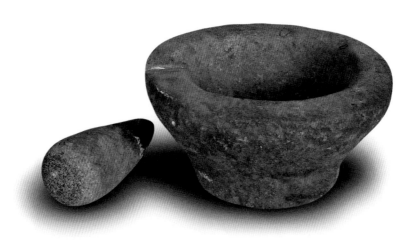

石研钵及杵

清

石质

钵：口外径 18.5 厘米，口内径 13.5 厘米，底径 12 厘米，通高 9.8 厘米

杵：长 12.5 厘米，直径 5 厘米

Stone Mortar and Pestle

Qing Dynasty

Stone

Mortar: Outer Diameter 18.5 cm/ Inner Diameter 13.5 cm/ Bottom Diameter 12 cm/ Height 9.8 cm

Pestle: Length 12.5 cm/ Diameter 5 cm

由黑色石料雕琢而成，表面粗糙。钵呈碗状，敞口，平底，壁较厚。杵呈圆棒状，一端粗，一端细。为制药工具，石质研钵可以使某些药材在研制时不与铜、铁等金属材料接触，避免发生化学反应。

中华医学会 / 上海中医药大学医史博物馆藏

The mortar and the pestle are made of black stone by grinding and chiseling. They have a rough surface. The mortar is shaped like a bowl with a flared mouth, a flat bottom, and a thick wall. The pestle looks like a round stick, with a thick end and a thin side. They were utilized for porphyrizing drug ingredients. Stone mortars could avoid chemical reactions by preventing some medicinal materials from contacting metals like copper and iron in drug preparation.

Preserved in Chinese Medical Association/ Museum of Chinese Medicine, Shanghai University of Traditional Chinese Medicine

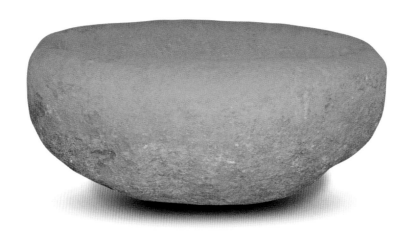

石药碾

清

石质

长 64 厘米，宽 31 厘米，高 29 厘米

Stone Medicine Crusher

Qing Dynasty

Stone

Length 64 cm/ Width 31 cm/ Height 29 cm

由整块砂岩雕琢而成。呈船形，中间有一碾
槽。为制药工具。陕西省西安市征集。

陕西医史博物馆藏

The crusher is made of a whole sandstone by
grinding and chiseling. It is shaped like a boat
with a mill groove in the middle of the crusher.
The crusher was a tool of medicine preparation.
It was collected in Xi'an City, Shaanxi Province.
Preserved in Shaanxi Museum of Medical History

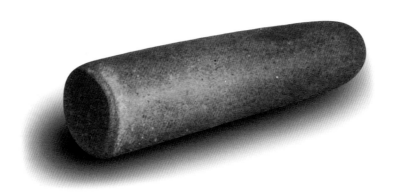

卵石药杵

清

石质

长 13.3 厘米，底径 4 厘米

Pebble Medicine Pestle

Qing Dynasty

Stone

Length 13.3 cm/ Bottom Diameter 4 cm

由整块黑褐色卵石制成，呈圆棒状，粗的一端较平，稍细的一端较圆。整体器形规整，有使用痕迹。为民间传世品，已经流传使用三世。

成都中医药大学中医药传统文化博物馆藏

The pestle is made of a whole dark brown pebble. It is shaped like a round stick. One end of the pestle is thick and flat while the other end is thin and round. On the surface of the well-structured pestle, there are some traces of using. It has already been handed down to three generations.

Preserved in Museum of Traditional Chinese Medicine Culture, Chengdu University of Traditional Chinese Medicine

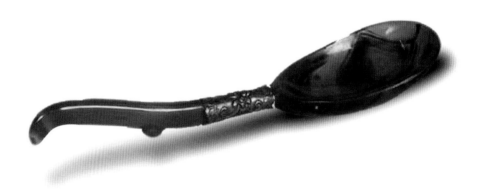

药勺

清

琥珀质

长 15.4 厘米，宽 3.3 厘米

Medicine Spoon

Qing Dynasty

Amber

Length 15.4 cm/ Width 3.3 cm

红褐色琥珀雕琢磨制而成，勺状，勺柄和勺部用金属连接。琥珀质地优良，全勺通体打磨光滑，加工工艺较好。制药工具。保存基本完好。

中华医学会 / 上海中医药大学医史博物馆藏

The spoon is made of reddish-brown amber by chiseling and grinding. The spoon handle and the body are connected with metal. The amber has a fine quality and a smooth surface. The processing technology of this spoon was good. The spoon was a tool of medicine preparation. The collection is still in good condition.

Preserved in Chinese Medical Association/ Museum of Chinese Medicine, Shanghai University of Traditional Chinese Medicine

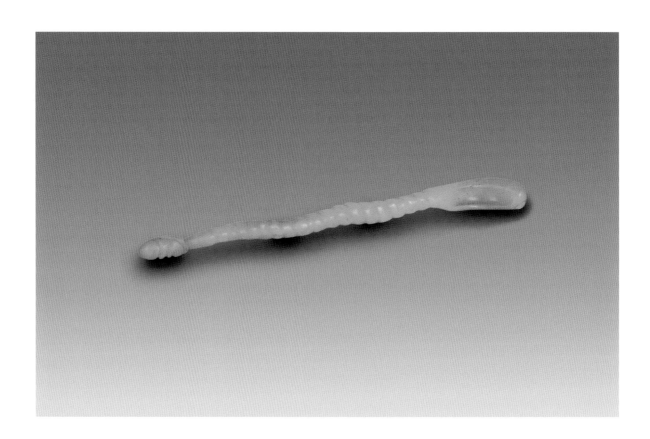

玉药勺

清

玉质

通长 13.05 厘米，勺宽 1 厘米，勺厚 0.9 厘米

Jade Medicine Spoon

Qing Dynasty

Jade

Length 13.05 cm/ Width 1 cm/ Thickness 0.9 cm

白玉制成。勺形，勺柄较长，有螺旋纹。为医用器具。1957 年入藏。

中华医学会 / 上海中医药大学医史博物馆藏

The spoon, made of white jade, has a long handle with spiral patterns. It was used as a medical appliance. The spoon was collected in 1957.

Preserved in Chinese Medical Association/ Museum of Chinese Medicine, Shanghai University of Traditional Chinese Medicine

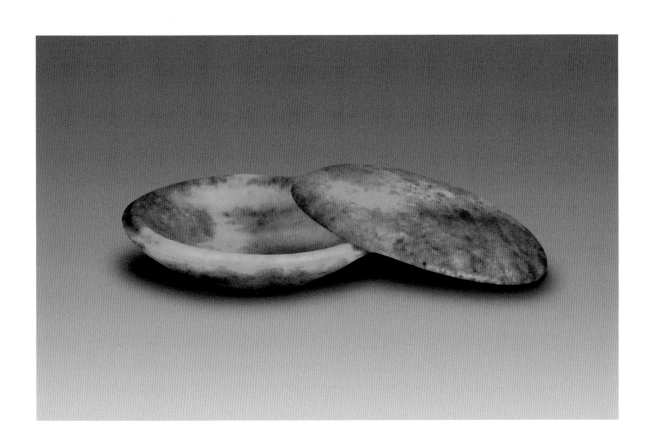

玉药盒

清

玉质

直径 5.36 厘米，厚 2 厘米

Jade Medicine Box

Qing Dynasty

Jade

Diameter 5.36 cm/ Thickness 2 cm

整体由玉料雕成，扁圆形。由盒和盖两部分组
成，扣合紧密，磨制精细。存药用。1956年入藏。

中华医学会 / 上海中医药大学医史博物馆藏

The medicine box, which is made of jade, is oblate
in shape. Its body and lid are buckled closely, which
shows the delicate grinding technique. It was used
for storing drugs. The box was collected in 1956.
Preserved in Chinese Medical Association/ Museum
of Chinese Medicine, Shanghai University of
Traditional Chinese Medicine

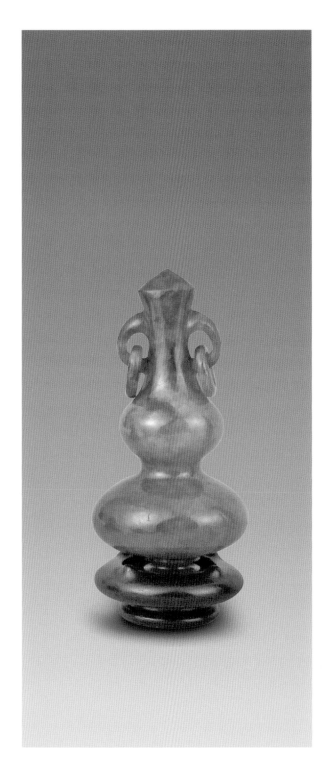

玉葫芦

清

玉质

上腹径 3.3 厘米，下腹径 4.4 厘米，腰径 1.8 厘米，
吊环直径 1.4 厘米，通高 8.6 厘米

Jade Gourd

Qing Dynasty

Jade

Upper Abdomen Diameter 3.3 cm/ Lower Abdomen
Diameter 4.4 cm/ Waist Diameter 1.8 cm/ Diameter
of the Ring 1.4 cm/ Height 8.6 cm

为深绿色玉质雕成，葫芦形，实心。葫芦颈部
两侧有耳，耳上垂环。雕工细腻，磨制光滑，
晶莹剔透，具较高观赏、收藏价值。为工艺品。
1954 年入藏。

中华医学会 / 上海中医药大学医史博物馆藏

The solid gourd is made of dark green jade. It is
shaped like a gourd with ears on both sides of
the neck. There are dangling rings on the ears.
The gourd is smooth, translucent and clear with
delicate carving technique. It has high values of
ornament and collection as an artware. The gourd
was collected in 1954.

Preserved in Chinese Medical Association/ Museum
of Chinese Medicine, Shanghai University of
Traditional Chinese Medicine

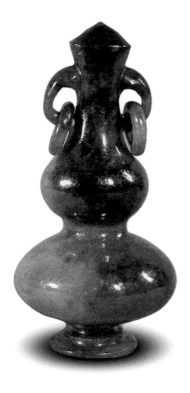

玉葫芦药瓶

清

玉质

底径 3 厘米，高 8 厘米

Gourd-shaped Jade Medicine Bottle

Qing Dynasty

Jade

Bottom Diameter 3 cm/ Height 8 cm

青色玉质雕成，葫芦形，上有盖。葫芦颈部两侧有耳，耳上垂环。雕工细腻，磨制光滑，晶莹剔透。内置药粉，可见是储药器具。

上海中医药博物馆藏

The bottle was carved out of green jade. It is shaped like a gourd and has a lid on the top. There are ears on both sides of the gourd. There are dangling rings on the ears. The gourd is smooth, translucent and clear with delicate carving technique. There are some drug powders in it. The bottle was used for storing drugs.

Preserved in Shanghai Museum of Traditional Chinese Medicine

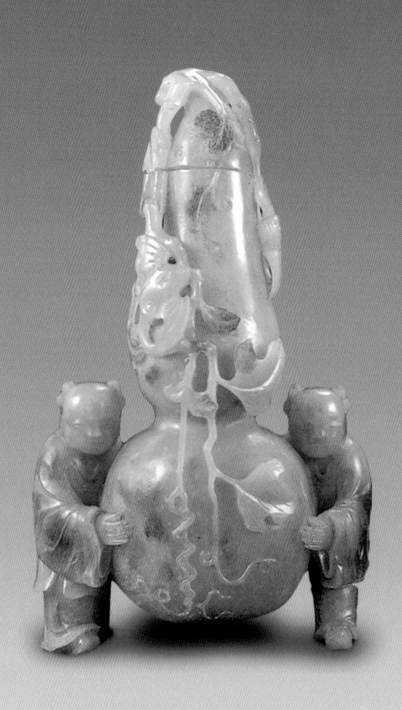

青玉童子葫芦瓶

清

玉质

底宽 10 厘米，通高 7.3 厘米

由整块青玉雕成。为带盖葫芦形瓶，中空，瓶外壁雕刻有两只趴伏在枝叶上相向的蝙蝠，瓶下部的两侧各有一头梳挽成双髻的童子呈双手抱瓶状。

河北博物院藏

Gourd-shaped Green Jade Bottle Held by Two Children

Qing Dynasty

Jade

Bottom Width 10 cm/ Height 7.3 cm

The bottle is made of a whole green jade. It is shaped like a hollow gourd with a lid. On the exterior wall of the bottle there are two crouching bats carved on the branches. On each lower side of the bottle is a child with double hair knots holding the bottle in both hands.

Preserved in Hebei Museum

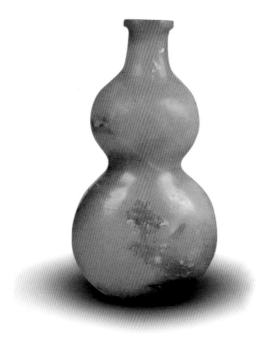

葫芦瓶

清

玉质

宽 6.7 厘米，通高 13.52 厘米，壁厚 3.1 厘米

Gourd-shaped Bottle

Qing Dynasty

Jade

Width 6.7 cm/ Height 13.52 cm/ Wall Thickness 3.1 cm

整体由白色玉料雕成。呈扁葫芦形，有口无盖，
口沿残。为艺术品。1957 年入藏。

中华医学会 / 上海中医药大学医史博物馆藏

The bottle was carved out of white jade. It is shaped
like an oblate gourd with a mouth but no lid. The
mouth rim is incomplete. As a work of art, it was
collected in 1957.

Preserved in Chinese Medical Association/ Museum
of Chinese Medicine, Shanghai University of
Traditional Chinese Medicine

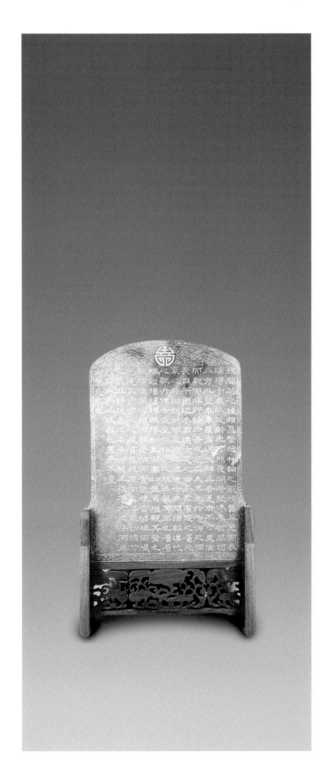

内廷《灵芝赋》青玉屏

清

玉质

宽 23 厘米，高 32 厘米，厚 1.1 厘米

Green Jade Screen with *Ling Zhi Fu*

Qing Dynasty

Jade

Width 23 cm/ Height 32 cm/ Thickness 1.1 cm

整体由青色玉料雕琢而成，方形。正面顶部
为半圆形，中间刻有篆书的"寿"字，左、
右刻镂以双钩蝙蝠，意为"福寿双全"。屏
体以隶书刻有乾隆皇帝所作《灵芝赋》。反
面用工笔双钩刻有灵芝和山石花卉，层缀相
交，均填以金粉。系清乾隆内廷供奉之物。

上海中医药博物馆藏

The square screen is made of a whole green
jade. The front top of the screen is semicircular
and the word "longevity" is engraved in seal
script in the middle. On both sides there are
hollowed bats, symbolizing blessing and longevity.
On the body of the screen is engraved in official
script a poem entitled *Ling Zhi Fu*(Inditement
of Ganoderma), written by Emperor Qianlong.
On the reverse side of the screen there are glossy
ganoderma, mountains and flowers engraved with
fine brushwork，which are all covered with gold
powders. The artifact was served in Emperor
Qianlong's inner court.
Preserved in Shanghai Museum of Traditional
Chinese Medicine

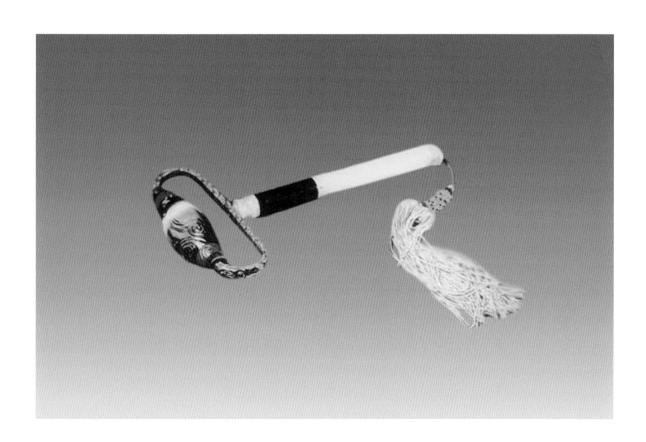

玉柄水晶按摩器

清

玉质

长约 30 厘米

Crystal Massager with Jade Handle

Qing Dynasty

Jade

Length 30 cm

按摩器呈滚筒状，器柄以水晶为之，按摩棒用玉石做成，套以金箍。在中国封建社会，皇帝及后妃自以为其体至贵，不可触摸，因而常以按摩器代之。可用于保健按摩。

故宫博物院藏

The massager is shaped like a cylinder. Its handle is made of jade. The crystal massager is decorated with gold hoop. In ancient China, servants were forbidden to touch the body of the emperor, the queen and concubines. Therefore, the servants used massagers when massaging them.

Preserved in The Palace Museum

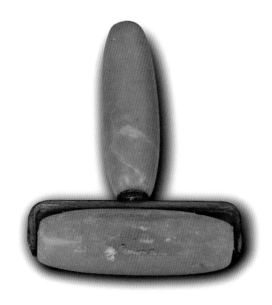

按摩器

清

玉石

滚筒：长 10 厘米，直径 3.3 厘米

柄：长 10 厘米，直径 3.3 厘米，通高 14.5 厘米

Massager

Qing Dynasty

Jade

Cylinder: Length 10 cm/ Diameter 3.3 cm

Handle: Length 10 cm/ Diameter 3.3 cm/ Height 14.5 cm

以青色玉料制成，滚筒状。用于按摩。山东省博物馆捐赠，1958 年入藏。

中华医学会 / 上海中医药大学医史博物馆藏

The massager, made of cyan jade, is shaped like a cylinder. It was utilized for massaging. It was donated by Shandong Museum and came in collection in 1958.

Preserved in Chinese Medical Association/ Museum of Chinese Medicine, Shanghai University of Traditional Chinese Medicine

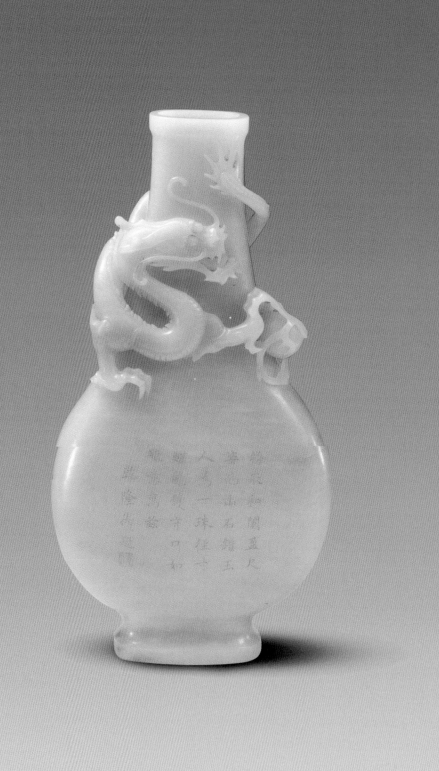

蟠龙纹白玉瓶

清

玉质

口径 5.2～6.2 厘米，足径 5.5～9.8 厘米，高 34.4 厘米

新疆和田玉雕琢而成。器体呈扁圆形，直口，高颈，扁圆腹，圈足。颈部镂雕骊龙蟠绕，护持骊珠。

山东博物馆藏

White Jade Bottle with Dragon Design

Qing Dynasty

Jade

Mouth Diameter 5.2–6.2 cm/ Bottom Diameter 5.5–9.8 cm/ Height 34.4 cm

The bottle was carved out of Hetian jade. The bottle has an oblate body, a vertical mouth, a tall neck, a flat belly, and a ring foot. The bottleneck is carved a winding dragon protecting a precious pearl.

Preserved in Shandong Museum

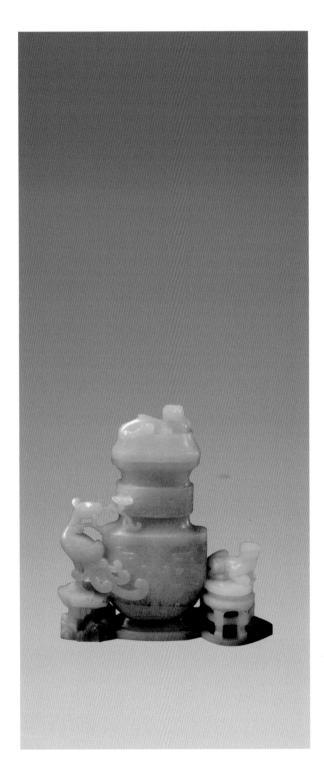

龙凤纹黄玉瓶

清

玉质

宽 12.4 厘米，厚 3.4 厘米，通高 14.4 厘米

Yellow Jade Bottle with Dragon and Phoenix Designs

Qing Dynasty

Jade

Width 12.4 cm/ Thickness 3.4 cm/ Height 14.4 cm

玉质晶莹，呈黄色，通体光亮。器体呈扁形，小口，细颈，扁腹，下接横座，左侧透雕一凤，右侧透雕一龙，上有盖，龙形钮。质料名贵，形制新颖，线条圆润。

山东博物馆藏

The bottle is made of translucent yellow jade. It has a flat body, a small mouth, a lid with a dragon-shaped knob, a narrow neck, and a flat belly. The bottle is connected with a stand carved with a phoenix on the left and one carved with a dragon on the right. The jade material is precious, the design is novel, and the lines are smooth.

Preserved in Shandong Museum

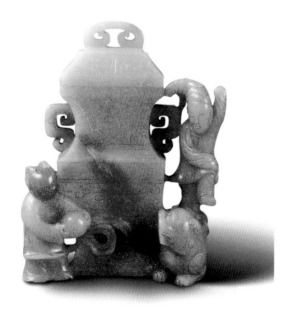

黄玉蕃人戏狮双耳玉盖瓶

清

玉质

宽 11.8 厘米，高 14.1 厘米

Yellow Jade Bottle with Two Ears, Jade Cover and Pattern of a Person of Minority Group Teasing a Lion

Ming Dynasty

Jade

Width 11.8 cm/ Height 14.1 cm

玉呈深黄色。瓶身刻兽面纹、蕉叶纹等，瓶左侧一蕃人呈舞蹈戏狮状，右侧一童子手持绣球与舞者对应。

天津艺术博物馆藏

The jade is dark yellow. The body of the bottle is carved with patterns of the beast's face and banana leaves. The left side of the bottle is carved with a person of the minority group dancing and teasing a lion. The right side of the bottle is carved with a boy holding a ball made of strips of silk.

Preserved in Tianjin Art Museum

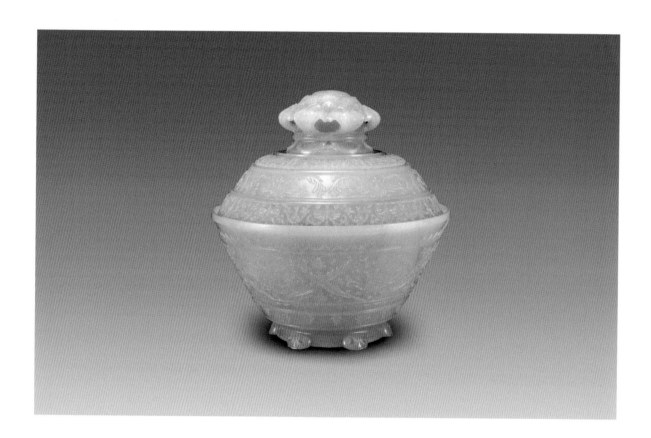

玉宝相花盖碗

清

玉质

口径 16.1 厘米，足径 8.6 厘米，高 16.5 厘米

Jade Tea Tureen with Rosette Designs

Qing Dynasty

Jade

Mouth Diameter 16.1 cm/ Foot Diameter 8.6 cm/ Height 16.5 cm

盖顶雕团"寿"字，足内刻隶书双行"乾隆年制"款。主体纹饰为宝相花。宝相花又称宝仙花，是以牡丹或莲花为本抽象而成，喻义"宝""仙"，盛行于隋唐。

故宫博物院藏

The top of its lid is carved into the shape of a Chinese word which means longevity. At the bottom of the tureen there are two-lined inscriptions engraved in official seal "Qian Long Nian Zhi" (made in Qianlong Reign). The main part of the tureen is decorated with rosette designs in the shape of peony or lotus, meaning treasure and immortality, respectively. The design was popular in the Sui and Tang Dynasties.

Preserved in The Palace Museum

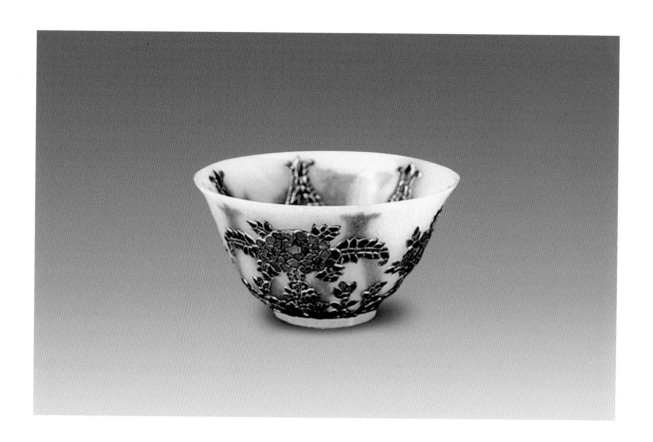

描金嵌宝石玉碗

清

玉质

口径 10.1 厘米，底径 4.8 厘米，高 6.5 厘米

Jade Bowl Inlaid with Gem and Gold-painted Designs

Qing Dynasty

Jade

Mouth Diameter 10.1 cm/ Bottom Diameter 4.8 cm/ Height 6.5 cm

玉呈青白色。碗敞口，矮圈足。碗腹为描金
嵌宝石的花草绿叶相拥的宝相花图案，内壁
为六组石榴纹。

山西博物院藏

The color of the jade bowl is cyan. The bowl
has a flared mouth and a short ring foot. The
body of the bowl is decorated with gold-painted
and intertwining flower designs. The interior
wall of the bowl is decorated with six sets of
pomegranate designs.

Preserved in Shanxi Museum

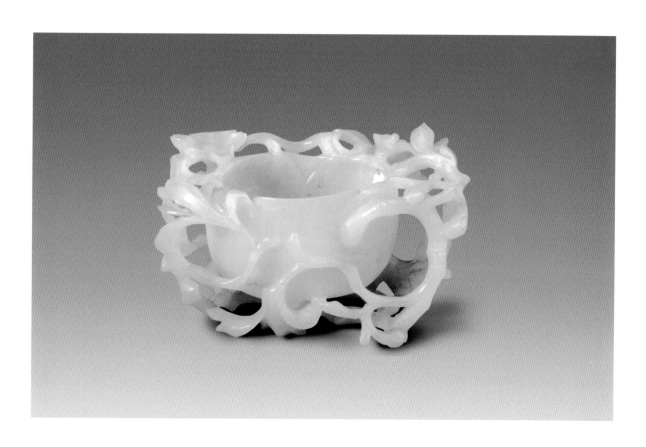

青玉百合花杯

清

玉质

长 11.2 厘米，高 5.5 厘米

Sapphire Cup with Lily Designs

Qing Dynasty

Jade

Length 11.2 cm/ Height 5.5 cm

青玉雕琢而成，玉质莹润。杯口呈椭圆形，

杯呈钵状。杯两侧镂孔较大，可作杯柄。

山西博物院藏

The cup, which was carved out of sapphire, is moisturized and translucent. The cup has an oval rim and a mortar-shaped body. The big hollowed sides of the cup were utilized as a handle.

Preserved in Shanxi Museum

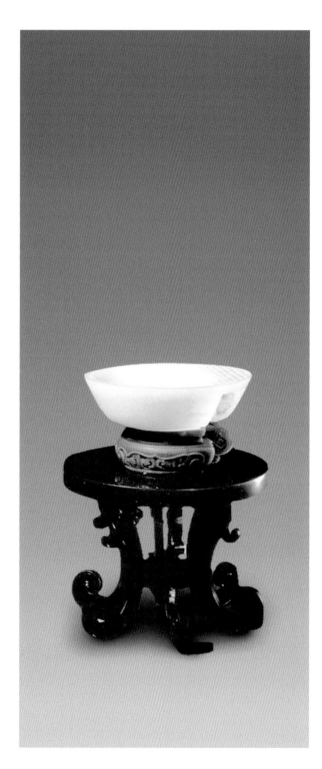

玉寿字洗

清

玉质

口径 13.5 厘米，足径 10 厘米，洗高 3.7 厘米，

通座架高 19 厘米

Jade Washing Basin

Qing Dynasty

Jade

Mouth Diameter 13.5 cm/ Foot Diameter 10 cm/

Basin Height 3.7 cm/ Holder Height 19 cm

洗由白玉雕琢而成，敞口，平底。器表为"寿"字、灵芝纹及几处半圆的如意头式的造型，体现了健康长寿、吉祥如意的主题，是传统吉祥题材的一种。

故宫博物院藏

The jade washing basin, carved out of white jade, has a flared mouth and a flat bottom. The surface of the basin is patterned with the word "longevity", ganoderma and several hemispherical ruyi, all of which embody the theme of good health, longevity and good luck. Preserved in The Palace Museum

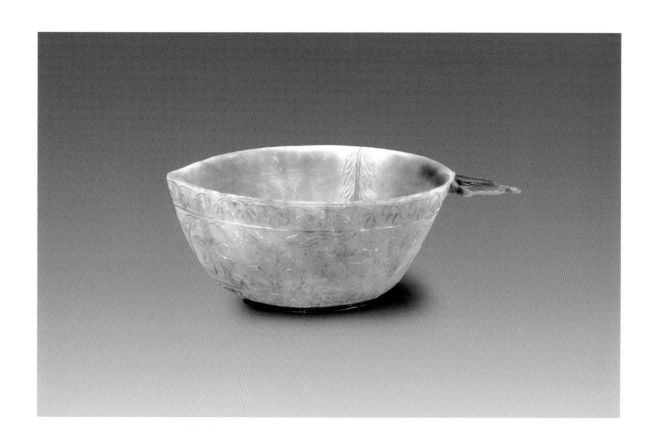

痕都斯坦玉洗

清

玉质

口长径 19.1 厘米，短径 16.7 厘米，足长径 9.2 厘米，短径 6.8 厘米，高 8.5 厘米

Hindustan Jade Basin

Qing Dynasty

Jade

Long Mouth Diameter 19.1 cm/ Short Mouth Diameter 16.7 cm/ Long Foot Diameter 9.2 cm/ Short Foot

Diameter 6.8 cm/ Height 8.5 cm

痕都斯坦玉雕成，敞口，一侧带流，平底。
器表阴刻花叶纹饰，纹饰中突出一叶为柄。
该器形体较大，器壁匀薄，显出加工难度。
痕都斯坦玉器即回教或伊斯兰玉器，在清代
宫廷中是非常名贵而特别的一种。

故宫博物院藏

The Hindustan jade basin was carved in patterns
of intaglio leaves, one of which serves as the
handle. It has a flared mouth, a side with a
spout, a flat bottom, and a big body. The wall
is evenly thin, which shows the difficulty of
processing. Hindustan jade, also called Islam
jade, was a special and rare type of jade in the
imperial court of the Qing Dynasty.

Preserved in The Palace Museum

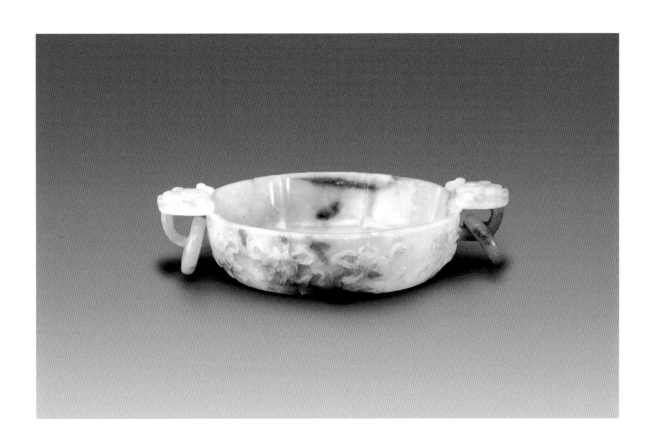

玉雕带环洗

清

玉质

长 20.5 厘米，直径 14.7 厘米

Jade Washing Basin with Rings

Qing Dynasty

Jade

Length 20.5 cm/ Diameter 14.7 cm

青玉雕成，有褐色沁斑。杯呈变形海棠式。

口稍撇，雕兽首双耳，颌下一长柄接于腹部。

山西博物院藏

The basin was carved out of gray jade. It has
some brown spots. The basin is shaped like
a distorted malus spectabilis with a slightly
extended mouth and ears carved with an
animal's head on both sides. A long handle
connects the mouth with the belly of the basin.
Preserved in Shanxi Museum

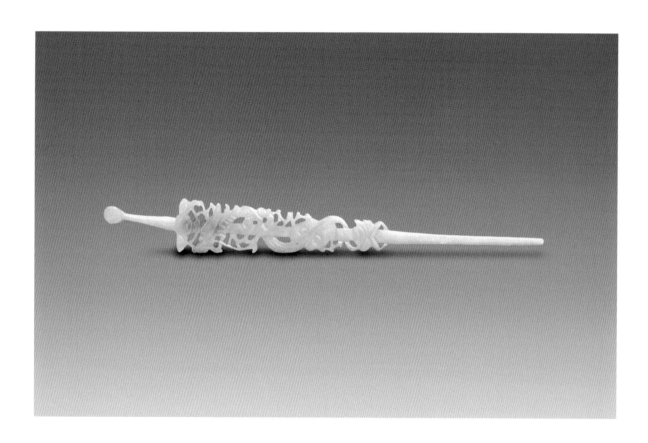

青玉簪

清

玉质

长 18.5 厘米

Gray Jade Hairpin

Qing Dynasty

Jade

Length 18.5 cm

青玉雕成。上部翘起，顶端扁圆如耳勺，中
部镂雕盘龙。簪头由粗渐细，光滑圆润。

山西博物院藏

The hairpin was carved out of gray jade. The
upper part of this hairpin is cocking up, with an
oblate top which looks like an ear spoon. The
middle part is carved with a hollowed winding
dragon. The head of the hairpin is tapered. The
hairpin is smooth and mellow.

Preserved in Shanxi Museum

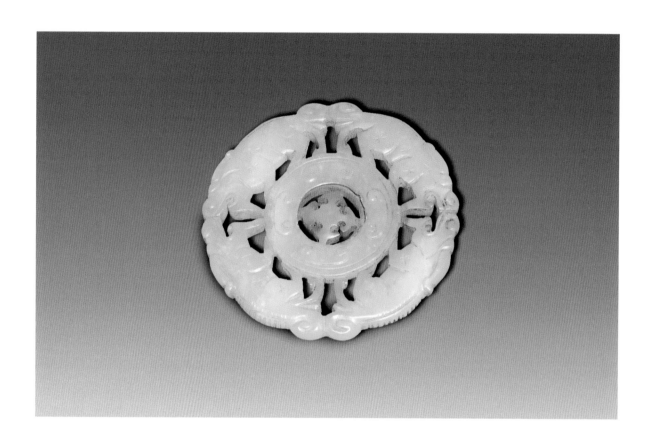

玉佩

清

玉质

直径 5.5 厘米，厚 0.5 厘米

Jade Pendant

Qing Dynasty

Jade

Diameter 5.5 cm/ Thickness 0.5 cm

白玉雕成。圆形，中心部有云纹活动钮，中间圆壁上刻四个云纹，外圈刻四只走兽，两两相对。为装饰品。陕西咸阳秦都区公安局移交。

陕西医史博物馆藏

The pendant, which is made of white jade, is round in shape. Its central part has a movable button with cloud designs. There are four cloud patterns on the wall of the central circle and two pairs of beasts on the outer ring. The pendant was a decoration. It was transferred by the Public Security Bureau of Qindu District of Xianyang City, Shaanxi Province.

Preserved in Shaanxi Museum of Medical History

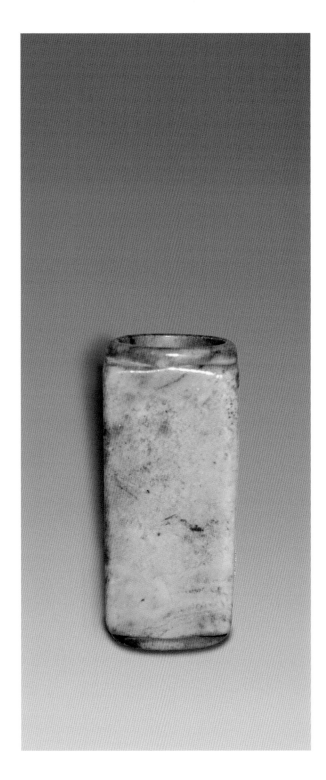

玉琮

清

玉质

口径 4 厘米，底径 3.7 厘米，高 9.5 厘米，重
291 克

Jade Cong

Qing Dynasty

Jade

Mouth Diameter 4 cm/ Bottom Diameter 3.7 cm/

Height 9.5 cm/ Weight 291 g

黄玉雕成。圆口，腹为长方体，圆平底。为
祭祀用品。

陕西医史博物馆藏

The jade cong was carved out of topaz. It has
a round mouth, a flat and round bottom, and a
cuboid belly. It was a sacrificial item.

Preserved in Shaanxi Museum of Medical History

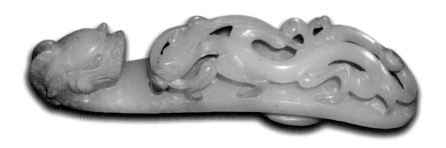

龙头螭纹玉带钩

清

玉质

长 12.2 厘米，宽 1.5～2.2 厘米

Jade Belt Hook with Chi Dragon Designs

Qing Dynasty

Jade

Length 12.2 cm/ Width 1.5–2.2 cm

白玉雕成。呈"S"状，一端为龙头，为母
子龙形动物浮雕图饰，背为蝉钮。为生活用具。
陕西省咸阳市秦都区公安局移交，1989 年入
藏，级别为二级。

陕西医史博物馆藏

The hook, which is made of white jade, is
S-shaped. One end is a dragon in relief, whose
back is a cicada-shaped button. The hook was
a utensil for daily use. It was transferred by
the Public Security Burean of Qindu District
of Xianyang City, Shaanxi province. It was
collected by the museum in 1989 and rated
Class 2.

Preserved in Shaanxi Museum of Medical History

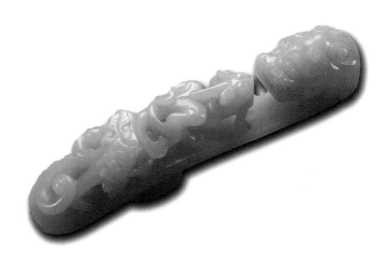

白玉龙纹带钩

清

玉质

长 12.8 厘米，宽 2.7 厘米，高 2.5 厘米

Jade Belt Hook with Dragon Designs

Qing Dynasty

Jade

Length 12.8 cm/ Width 2.7 cm/ Height 2.5 cm

白玉雕成，玉质晶莹。带钩头部为立雕龙首，正面雕一螭与龙对视，背面有一圆钮。

常州博物馆藏

The crystal-clear belt hook was carved out of white jade. The head of this hook is carved as a dragon's head. On the front side is a chi dragon facing the dragon. There is a round button on the back side of the hook.

Preserved in Changzhou Museum

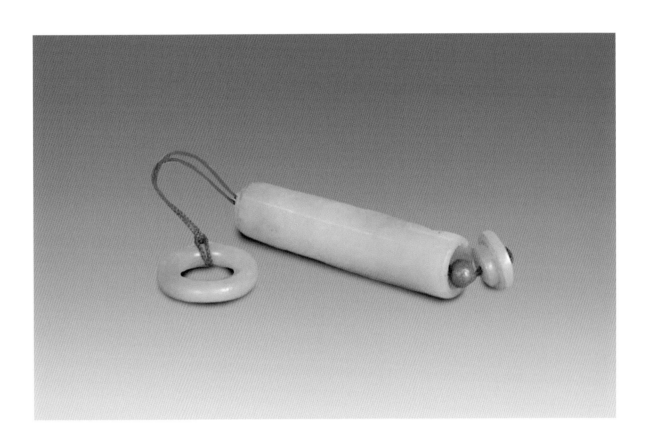

避瘟香珠筒

清

玉质

通长 6.95 厘米，筒外径 1.45 厘米，筒壁厚 0.25 厘米

Aromatic Bead Cylinder as Protection Against Diseases

Qing Dynasty

Jade

Length 6.95 cm/ Outer Diameter 1.45 cm/ Wall Thickness 0.25 cm

白玉雕成。圆筒形，一端有盖，盖上系香珠7粒；
另一端配有一环，也为白玉所制。为医疗用具。
1954 年入藏。

中华医学会 / 上海中医药大学医史博物馆藏

The collection, which is made of white jade, is
cylindrical. On one end of it there is a lid with seven
aromatic beads. On the other end there is a ring
of white jade. The artifact, which was used for
medical purposes, was collected by the museum
in 1954.

Preserved in Chinese Medical Association/ Museum
of Chinese Medicine, Shanghai University of
Traditional Chinese Medicine

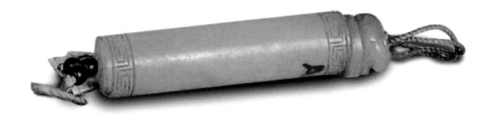

避瘟香珠筒

清

玉质

通长 6.2 厘米，筒外径 1.15 厘米，筒壁厚 0.25 厘米

Aromatic Bead Cylinder as Protection Against Diseases

Qing Dynasty

Jade

Length 6.2 cm/ Outer Diameter 1.15 cm/ Wall Thickness 0.25 cm

白玉雕成。圆筒形，一端有盖，盖上有兽钮。
盖与筒身由一细绳串联。为医疗用具。1954 年
入藏。

中华医学会 / 上海中医药大学医史博物馆藏

The collection, which is made of white jade, is
cylindrical. On one end of it there is a lid with a
beast-shaped button. A string ties the lid with the
body. The cylinder, which was used for medical
purposes, was collected by the museum in 1954.
Preserved in Chinese Medical Association/ Museum
of Chinese Medicine, Shanghai University of
Traditional Chinese Medicine

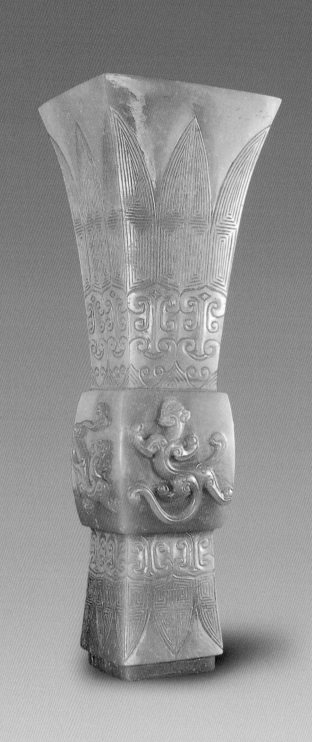

青玉觚

清

玉质

纵径 9 厘米，横径 7.3 厘米，高 24.9 厘米

青玉雕成。方形。喇叭形侈口，束腰，高圈足外撇。外壁饰蝉纹和几何纹，中间凸起的四周有浅浮雕蟠螭纹。

河北博物院藏

Sapphire Gu-vessel

Qing Dynasty

Jade

Vertical Diameter 9 cm/ Horizontal Diameter 7.3 cm/ Height 24.9 cm

The collection, which was carved out of sapphire, is rectangular. The Gu-vessel has a wide trumpet-shaped mouth, a narrow waist, and a high ring foot extended outwards. The exterior wall is decorated with geometric and cicada patterns while the protruded middle part is surrounded by dragon designs in bas-relief.

Preserved in Hebei Museum

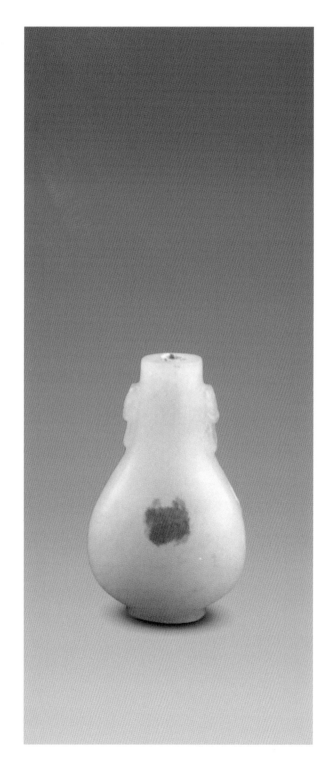

白玉鼻烟壶

清

玉质

口外径 1.1 厘米，底长径 1.5 厘米，底短径

1.3 厘米，通高 4.65 厘米，重 26 克

White Jade Snuff Bottle

Qing Dynasty

Jade

Mouth Diameter 1.1 cm/ Bottom Long Diameter

1.5 cm/ Bottom Short Diameter 1.3 cm/ Height 4.65 cm/

Weight 26 g

白玉雕成。扁壶状，直口，鼓腹，平底，圈足。
为盛装鼻烟的容器。

广东中医药博物馆藏

The bottle is made of white jade. It is shaped
like a flat bottle with a straight mouth, a bulged
belly, a flat bottom, and a ring foot. It was used
for storing snuff.

Preserved in Guangdong Chinese Medicine Museum

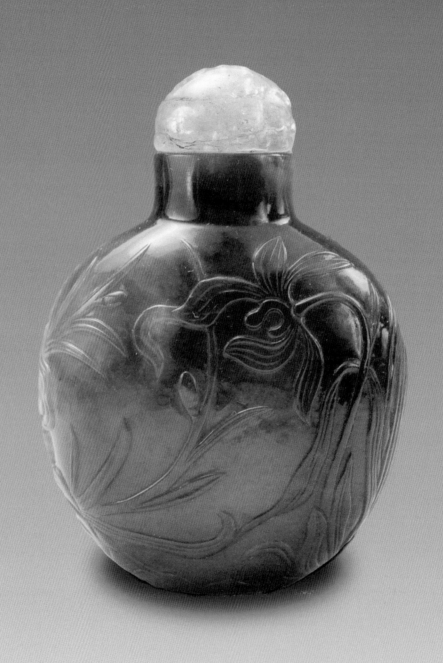

雕花翠烟壶

清

玉质

口径 1.8 厘米，底径 1.7～3.1 厘米，通高 5.3 厘米

葱绿色玉料雕成，翠质晶莹。小圆口，矮颈，扁圆腹，椭圆形底且内凹。通体浮雕花卉，山石上长出灵芝、兰草，花叶交错，生机盎然。

烟台市博物馆藏

Carved Green Jade Snuff Bottle

Qing Dynasty

Jade

Mouth Diameter 1.8 cm/ Bottom Diameter 1.7−3.1 cm/ Height 5.3 cm

The bottle was carved out of green jade. The jade is crystal-clear. The bottle has a round mouth, a short neck, a short round belly, and a dented oval bottom, The whole body of this bottle was carved with flowers and plants in relief. Ganodermas and fragrant thoroughworts grow out of the hillstones, which presents a picture full of life.

Preserved in Yantai Museum

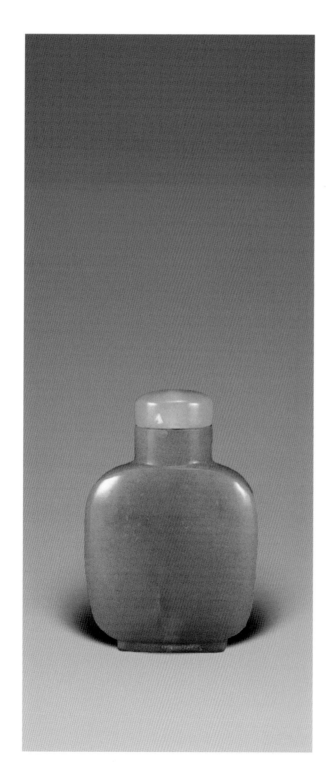

玛瑙扁烟壶

清

玉质

口径 2.6 厘米，高 4.4 厘米

Agate Snuff Bottle

Qing Dynasty

Jade

Diameter 2.6 cm/ Height 4.4 cm

黄色玛瑙雕成。扁壶状，直口带盖，长颈，腹部近方形，平底，圈足。清代用于鼻烟壶的材料很多，有玻璃、玉、翡翠、玛瑙、水晶、珐琅、陶瓷、青金石、竹木、象牙等，尤以乾隆时期最为繁荣。

故宫博物院藏

The collection is made of yellow agate. It is shaped like a flat bottle with a vertical mouth, a lid, a long neck, a square belly, a flat bottom, and a ring foot. In the Qing Dynasty snuff bottles were made of many materials such as glass, jade, emerald, agate, crystal, enamel, porcelain, lapis, bamboo, and ivory. Snuff bottles enjoyed the greatest prosperity in Qianlong Period.

Preserved in The Palace Museum

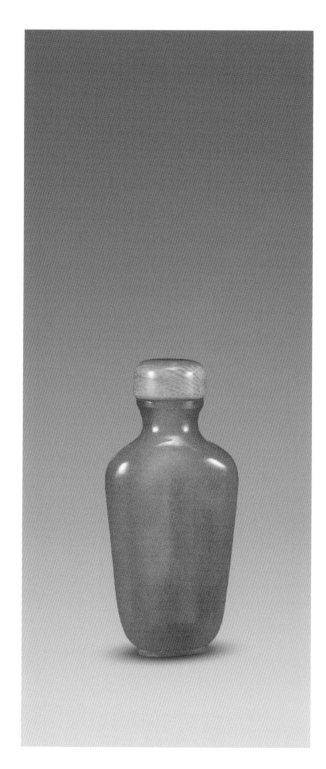

玛瑙烟壶

清

玉质

口径 1.5 厘米，高 5.9 厘米

Agate Snuff Bottle

Qing Dynasty

Jade

Mouth Diameter 1.5 cm/ Height 5.9 cm

黄色玛瑙雕琢而成。器形较高，侈口，带盖，斜腹内收，平底，圈足。鼻烟壶的盖下一般连有牙匙，以方便取用。清代鼻烟壶随着制作材料的增多，器型和装饰图案日趋复杂，表现题材多是山川、树木、吉祥花卉和神话传说等，光素无纹的并不多见。

故宫博物院藏

The bottle is made of yellow agate. It is tall with a wide mouth, a lid, an oblique abdomen, a flat bottom, and a ring foot. There is a tooth spoon under the lid, which makes using convenient. As snuff bottles were made of an increasing number of materials in the Qing Dynasty, the shape and decoration patterns of the bottles became more complex. As most of the themes were landscape, trees, auspicious flowers and legends, this type of smooth and plain snuff bottle was rarely seen.

Preserved in The Palace Museum

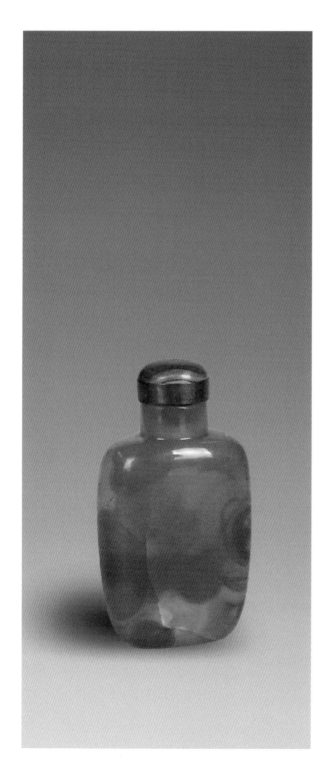

玛瑙烟壶

清

玉质

宽 3.25 厘米，厚 1.7 厘米，通高 6.55 厘米

Agate Snuff Bottle

Qing Dynasty

Jade

Width 3.25 cm/ Thickness 1.7 cm/ Height 6.55 cm

黄色玛瑙雕成。扁瓶状，直口带盖，腹部近方形，平底。该藏用于储存鼻烟粉，瓶盖连一小匙，以便存取粉末。1958 年入藏。

中华医学会 / 上海中医药大学医史博物馆藏

The collection is made of yellow agate. It is shaped like a flat bottle with a vertical mouth, a lid, a square belly, and a flat bottom. It was used for storing snuff powders. There is a spoon linked with the bottle lid, which makes using convenient. The bottle was collected by the museum in 1958.

Preserved in Chinese Medical Association/ Museum of Chinese Medicine, Shanghai University of Traditional Chinese Medicine

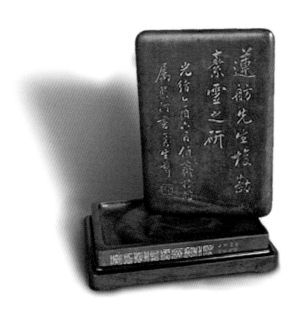

陈莲舫校勘砚

清

石质

长 15.9 厘米，宽 10.8 厘米，厚 2.9 厘米

Chen Lianfang's Collating Inkstone

Qing Dynasty

Stone

Length 15.9 cm/ Width 10.8 cm/ Thickness 2.9 cm

该砚台为清代医学家陈莲舫校勘砚。黑色石材制成，方形。砚台边款篆刻"莲舫先生校勘素灵之砚""乙酉初秋伯斋题赠"字样。砚配有红木套盒，盒盖刻有"莲舫先生校勘素灵之研""光绪乙酉六月伯斋持赠"等字样。陈莲舫，清代医家，世医业，少习儒。1900 年前后悬壶沪上，曾创办上海医会，先后五进宫城为帝治病。善治杂病，喜论医理。弟子众达二三百人，门人辑有《陈莲舫医案秘抄》。1958 年入藏。

中华医学会 / 上海中医药大学医史博物馆藏

This square inkstone, which is made of black stone, was owned by Chen Lianfang, a health expert in the Qing Dynasty. Its one side is inscribed with the owner of the inkstone and the time and place of inscription. A red sandalwood box that goes with the inkstone contains the same information on its lid. Chen Lianfang started his career in around 1900 and founded Shanghai Medical Association. He went to the imperial palace in Beijing to treat the emperor five times. He was an expert in medical theory and had as many as two or three hundred disciples, who compiled the book *Chen Lian Fang Yi An Mi Chao* (A Collection of Chen Lianfang's Medical Cases). This inkstone was collected by the museum in 1958.

Preserved in Chinese Medical Association/ Museum of Chinese Medicine, Shanghai University of Traditional Chinese Medicine

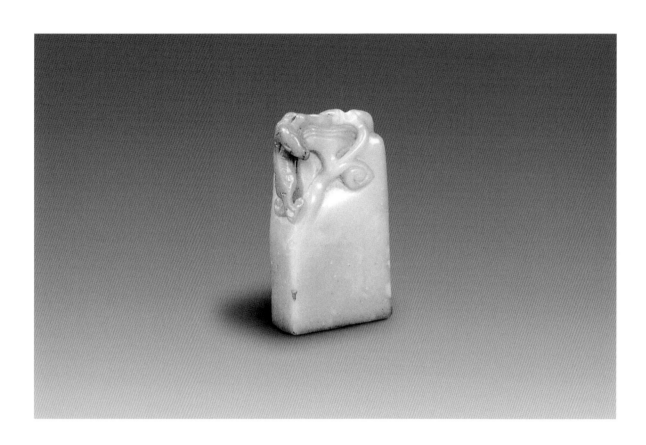

张查山用印

清

石质

长 3 厘米，宽 1.2 厘米，高 5.5 厘米

Seal Used by Zhang Chashan

Qing Dynasty

Stone

Length 3 cm/ Width 1.2 cm/ Height 5.5 cm

黄色细腻石料雕成。方形，印钮呈伏兽形。
印文为"张查山鉴藏图书印"，以元朱文入
印，精细工稳。为清代医学家张查山所用印
章。左图为其印蜕。张查山，名华，华亭人，
通医术，工诗文，善绘画。

上海中医药博物馆藏

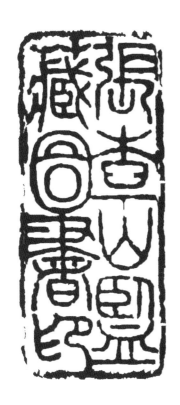

The seal was used by Zhang Chashan, a medical scientist in the Qing Dynasty. It was carved out of fine yellow stone. It is square with a crouching beast-shaped knob. The seal is inscribed with words indicating its owner. The picture on the left is the moulage of the seal. Zhang Chashan had a good knowledge of medicine, could compose poems and prose, and was good at painting.

Preserved in Shanghai Museum of Traditional Chinese Medicine

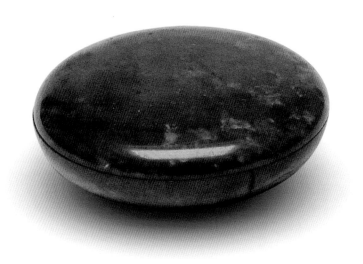

印砚

近代

石质

直径 7 厘米，高 4.5 厘米

Inkstone

Modern Times

Stone

Diameter 7 cm/ Height 4.5 cm

该藏由黑色细腻石料制成，呈圆饼形，制作规整，表面有光泽。由民间征集。

　　成都中医药大学中医药传统文化博物馆藏

The inkstone, which is made of fine black stone, is shaped like a round cake with a glossy surface. The inkstone was collected from a private owner.

Preserved in Museum of Traditional Chinese Medicine Culture, Chengdu University of Traditional Chinese Medicine

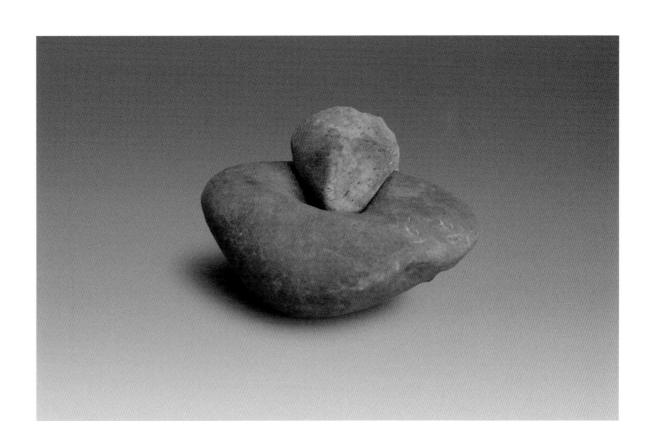

石臼

近代

石质

臼：直径 14 厘米，底径 10 厘米，高 12 厘米，重 3600 克

Stone Mortar and Pestle

Modern Times

Stone

Mortar: Diameter 14 cm/ Bottom Diameter 10 cm/ Height 12 cm/ Weight 3,600 g

臼和杵均为自然石块稍经加工而成。臼呈鼓
形，表面有一凹坑。杵为尖头卵石形。生产
生活器具，也可用于捣药。

陕西医史博物馆藏

The pestle and the mortar are made of natural
stone, The drum-shaped mortar has a dented
surface. The pestle is oval with a pointed end.
The collection was a tool for daily household
use and production. It could also be used to
smash medicine.

Preserved in Shaanxi Museum of Medical History

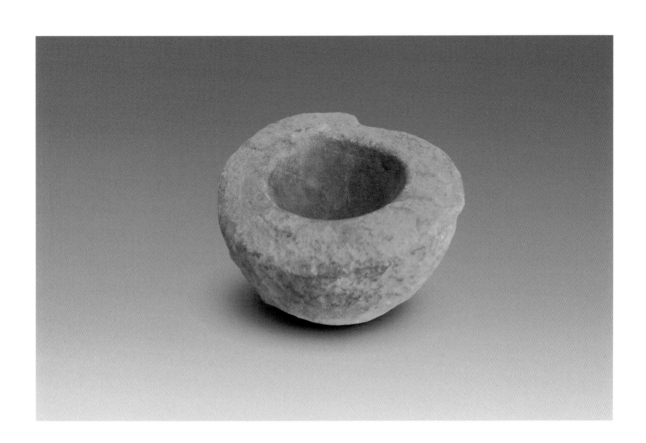

石臼

近代

石质

口外径 21 厘米，口内径 11 厘米，底径 14 厘米，高 9 厘米，臼窝深 5.5 厘米，重 6200 克

Stone Mortar

Modern Times

Stone

Mouth Outer Diameter 21 cm/ Mouth Inner Diameter 11 cm/ Bottom Diameter 14 cm/ Height 9 cm/

Depth 5.5 cm/ Weight 6,200 g

为自然石块稍经加工而成。呈半球形，表面有一凹坑。生产生活器具，也可用于捣药。

陕西医史博物馆藏

The mortar, which is made of natural stone, is hemispherical. There is a pit on the surface. The mortar was a tool for daily household use and production. It could also be used to smash medicine.

Preserved in Shaanxi Museum of Medical History

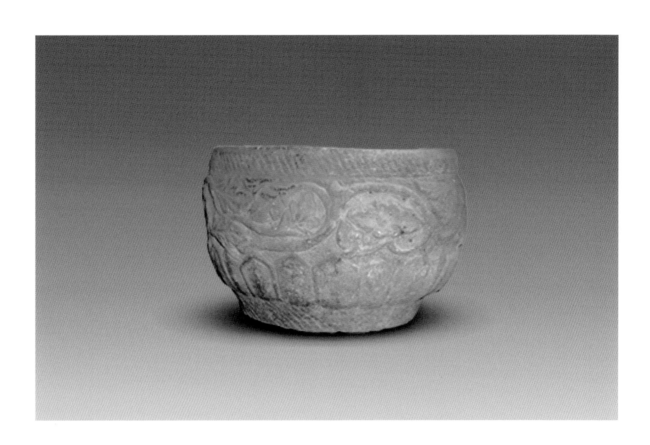

石臼

近代

石质

外径 41 厘米，内径 28 厘米，通高 28 厘米，臼深 14 厘米

Stone Mortar

Modern Times

Stone

Outer Diameter 41 cm/ Inner Diameter 28 cm/ Height 28 cm/ Depth 14 cm

圆口，平沿，鼓腹，平底。上腹一圈浮雕，
下腹一圈花瓣图。为生活器具、制药工具。
陕西省澄城县征集。

陕西医史博物馆藏

The mortar has a round mouth, a flat edge, a
bulged belly, and a flat bottom. There is a circle
of relief on the midsection and a circle of flower
petal designs in the lower part. The mortar was
used as a daily household tool for preparing
medicine. It was collected in Chengcheng
County, Shaanxi Province.

Preserved in Shaanxi Museum of Medical History

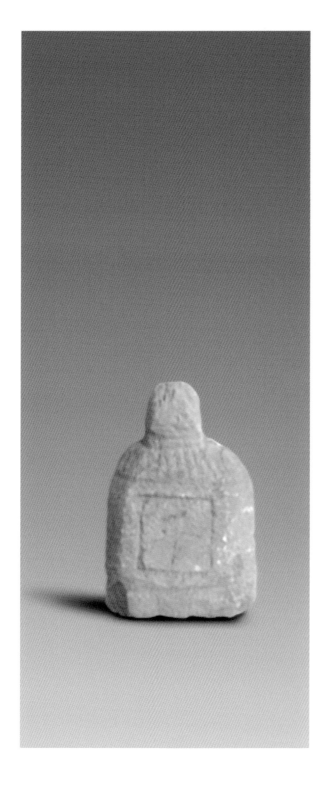

石镇

近代

石质

上宽 10 厘米，底宽 11 厘米，通高 25 厘米，重 9000 克

Stone Weight

Modern Times

Stone

Upper Width 10 cm/ Bottom Width 11 cm/ Height 25 cm/ Weight 9,000 g

砂岩石块雕琢而成。四棱形，石镇锤上刻有

"公平秤"字样。为文房、药店用具。

陕西医史博物馆藏

The prismatic weight was carved out of sandstone.
It is inscribed with three words "Gong Ping
Cheng" (fair scales). The collection was used in
the study or the drugstore.
Preserved in Shaanxi Museum of Medical History

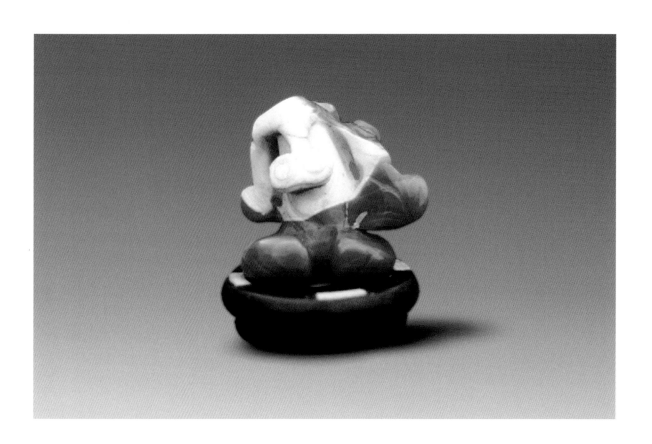

红玛瑙雕刻灵芝

近代

玉质

长 5.9 厘米，宽 4 厘米，通高 6.5 厘米，重 124 克

Red Agate-carved Ganoderma

Modern Times

Jade

Length 5.9 cm/ Width 4 cm/ Height 6.5 cm/ Weight 124 g

由玛瑙雕刻的艺术品，呈灵芝状，红白相间。
用于装饰。

广东中医药博物馆藏

The red and white collection is a piece of artistic work. It is made of agate and shaped like a ganoderma. It was used for decoration.

Preserved in Guangdong Chinese Medicine Museum

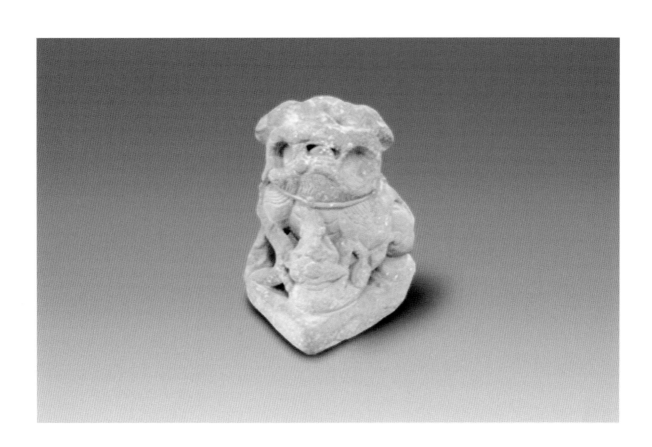

药兽

民国时期

石质

高 24 厘米

Medicine Beast

Republican Period

Stone

Height 24 cm

由整块砂岩雕琢而成。形似狮子，昂首，张口，立于方形底座上。传说为药王采药时所带的宠物，能帮助辨识药物，在以前四川的药铺中很常见，由民间征集。

成都中医药大学中医药传统文化博物馆藏

The collection is made of a whole block of sandstone. It is shaped like a lion standing on the square base with its head holding high and its mouth wide open. It is said that the King of Medicine usually took the pet to help him identify medicinal herbs when he went out gathering herbs. This type of stone beast used to be common in drugstores in Sichuan Province. It was collected from a private owner.

Preserved in Museum of Traditional Chinese Medicine Culture, Chengdu University of Traditional Chinese Medicine

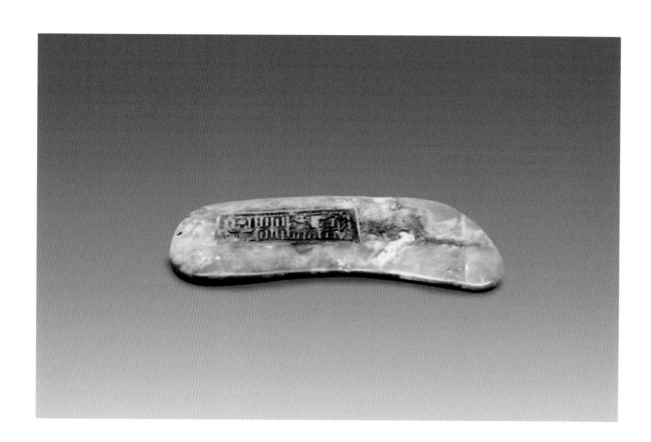

刮痧器

民国时期

玉质

长 12 厘米，宽 5 厘米

Scraping Device

Republican Period

Jade

Length 12 cm/ Width 5 cm

褐色玉料雕成。钺形，一端有小圆孔，为穿绳系带之用。器物一面有"杏林春暖"四字铭文。利用玉的莹润，再辅以麻油等物，在患者胸背、肘窝等部位刮痧，常可使患者周身轻松，舒适，病症减轻。此为一件精致的医用器具，保存完好。由民间征集。

成都中医药大学中医药传统文化博物馆藏

The hatchet-shaped scraping device was carved out of brown jade. On its one side there is a small round hole for lacing. The device is inscribed with four words. Scraping a patient's chest, back or cubital fossa by making use of the natural smoothness of jade and sesame oil can produce relaxing and symptom-alleviating effects. The well-preserved artifact is an exquisite medical device. It was collected from a private owner.

Preserved in Museum of Traditional Chinese Medicine Culture, Chengdu University of Traditional Chinese Medicine

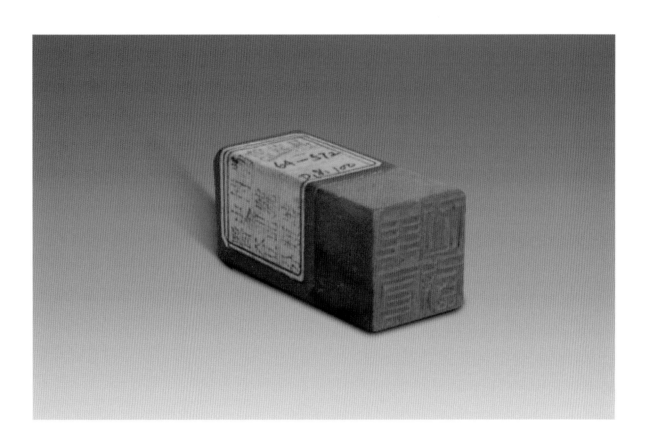

"巢凤初藏"章

近现代

石质

边长 2.03 厘米，高 4.4 厘米

Seal Collected by Chao Fengchu

Modern Times

Stone

Length 2.03 cm/ Height 4.4 cm

细腻石料雕成。长方体形，印文为"巢凤初藏"，可见为巢凤初私人收藏章。巢凤初，字崇山，武进孟河人。清代医家，精医术，善内、外科，门人众多。晚年号卧猿老人。1964 年入藏。

中华医学会 / 上海中医药大学医史博物馆藏

The cuboid seal was carved out of fine stone. It is inscribed with words "Chao Feng Chu Cang" (collected by Chao Fengchu), indicating that it was a private collection of Chao Fengchu, also named Chongshan. Chao Fengchu, a famous medical scientist in the Qing Dynasty, was an expert in both internal medicine and surgery. Therefore, he had many disciples. His assumed name Woyuan Laoren during his later years. The seal was collected in 1964.

Preserved in Chinese Medical Association/ Museum of Chinese Medicine, Shanghai University of Traditional Chinese Medicine

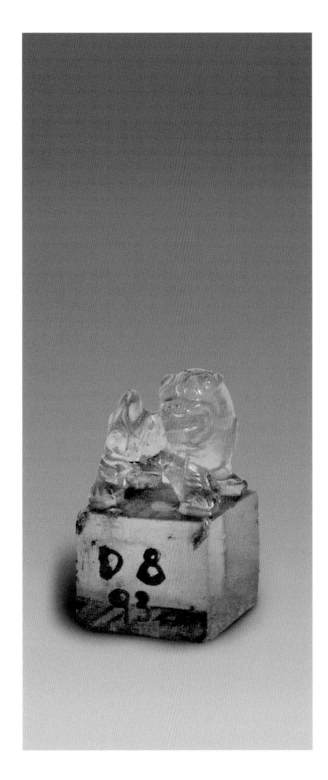

葛耘石所用闲章

近现代

玉质

边长 3.36 厘米，高 5.86 厘米

Seal Used by Ge Yunshi

Modern Times

Jade

Length 3.36 cm/ Height 5.86 cm

水晶雕成。方形，印钮为一站立狮子。为闲章，

印面为篆体白文，内容及葛耘石详情待考。

1961 年入藏。

中华医学会 / 上海中医药大学医史博物馆藏

The square seal was carved out of crystal. The
top part of the button is shaped like a standing
lion. It was an unofficial personal seal. Its surface
is carved in seal script. The content and Ge Yunshi
need to be studied. The seal was collected in 1961.
Preserved in Chinese Medical Association/ Museum
of Chinese Medicine, Shanghai University of
Traditional Chinese Medicine

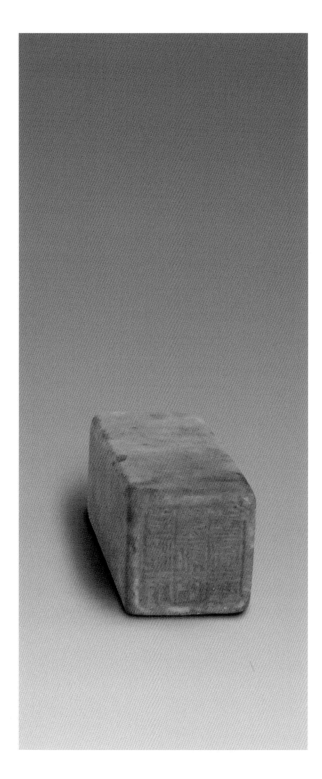

上海市医师公会图章

近现代

石质

边长 2.1 厘米，高 4.18 厘米

Seal of Shanghai Physicians' Association

Modern Times

Stone

Length 2.1 cm/ Height 4.18 cm

该藏为上海市医师公会图章。印章为长方体，印面正方形，字迹模糊不清。上海市医师公会原名上海医师公会，为蔡禹门、庞京周、汪企张、余云岫、徐乃礼等发起，于民国十四年十一月一日成立，下设学术演讲和民众卫生等专门委员会。会址在西藏路545号上海时疫医院内。该会于1951年解散。1955年入藏。

中华医学会/上海中医药大学医史博物馆藏

The collection was the seal of Shanghai Physicians' Association. The body of the seal is cuboid and the stamped side is square with indistinct words on it. Shanghai Physicians' Association was initiated by Cai Yumen, Pang Jingzhou, Wang Qizhang, Yu Yunxiu, and Xu Naili. It was founded on November 1, 1925. Under its administration there were several specialized committees such as the Academic Speech Committee and the Public Health Committee. The site of the association was in Shanghai Epidemic Hospital on the Tibet Road, No. 545, The association was dismissed in 1951. The seal was collected in 1955.

Preserved in Chinese Medical Association/ Museum of Chinese Medicine, Shanghai University of Traditional Chinese Medicine

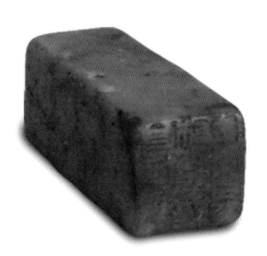

上海市医师公会经济委员石质方章

近现代

石质

长 1.4 厘米，宽 1.4 厘米，高 3.7 厘米

Stone Seal of Economy Committee Member of Shanghai Physicians' Association

Modern Times

Stone

Length 1.4 cm/ Width 1.4 cm/ Height 3.7 cm

该藏为上海市医师公会经济委员公章。印章为长方体，印面正方形，朱文刻"上海市医师公会经济委员印"，不留边框。上海市医师公会原名上海医师公会，为蔡禹门、庞京周、汪企张、余云岫、徐乃礼等发起，于 1952 年 11 月 1 日成立的西医职业团体，下设有编辑、学术演讲和民众卫生等专门委员会。会址在西藏路 545 号上海时疫医院内。发行《新医于社会》等刊物。该会于 1951 年解散。会员一度由 80 人增至 3208 人。1955 年入藏。

中华医学会 / 上海中医药大学医史博物馆藏

The collection was the seal of Economy Committee Member of Shanghai Physicians' Association. The body of the seal is cuboid and the stamped side is square with words carved in relief on it "ShangHai Shi Yi Shi Gong Hui Jing Ji Wei Yuan Yin" (Seal of Economy Committee Member of Shanghai Physicians' Association). Shanghai Physicians' Association was initiated by Cai Yumen, Pang Jingzhou, Wang Qizhang, Yu Yunxiu, and Xu Naili. It was founded on November 1, 1925. Under its administration there were several specialized committees such as the Editors' Committee, the Academic Speech Committee, and the Public Health Committee. The site of the association was in Shanghai Epidemic Hospital on the Tibet Road, No. 545. Its main publication was *New Medicine and the Society*. The association was dismissed in 1951. The number of its member once reached 3,208 from 80. The seal was collected in 1955.

Preserved in Chinese Medical Association/ Museum of Chinese Medicine, Shanghai University of Traditional Chinese Medicine

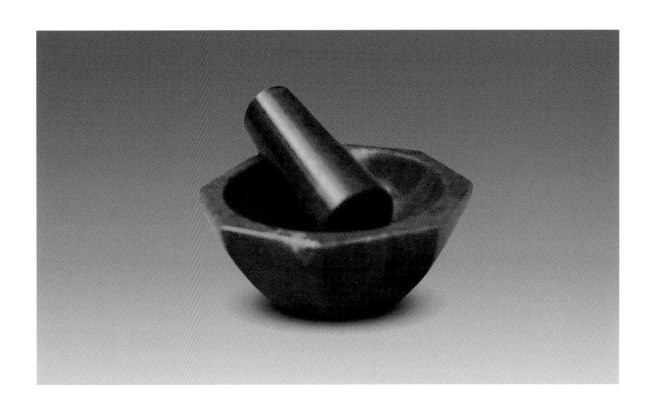

研钵

近现代

石质

钵：口径 10.7 厘米，底径 4.9 厘米，通高 4 厘米

杵：长 7.7 厘米

Mortar and Pestle

Modern Times

Stone

Mortar: Mouth Diameter 10.7 cm/ Bottom Diameter 4.9 cm/ Height 4 cm

Pestle: Length 7.7 cm

赭红色天然石料加工制成，外呈八角形，内呈
圆钵形，敞口，平底。通体磨光。配圆柱形杵。
制作精细，造型美观。1957 年入藏。

中华医学会 / 上海中医药大学医史博物馆藏

The mortar, which is made of natural reddish stone, is octagon-shaped outside and bowl-shaped inside. It has a flared mouth, a flat bottom, and a polished body. A cylindrical pestle goes with the mortar. The artifact was delicately made and looks artistic. It was collected by the museum in 1957.

Preserved in Chinese Medical Association/ Museum of Chinese Medicine, Shanghai University of Traditional Chinese Medicine

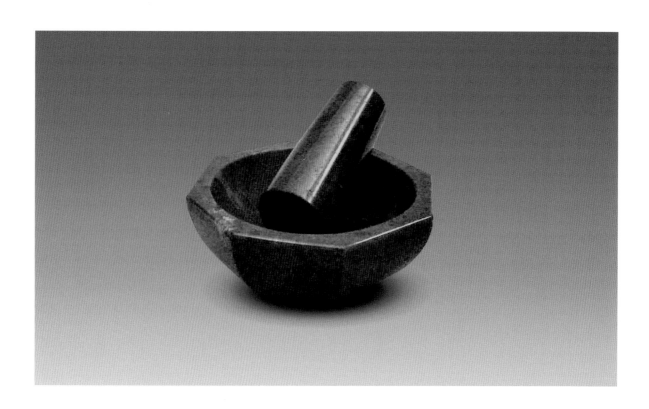

研钵

近现代

石质

钵：口径 10.7 厘米，通高 4 厘米

杵：长 7.7 厘米

Mortar and Pestle

Modern Times

Stone

Mortar: Diameter 10.7 cm/ Height 4 cm

Pestle: Length 7.7 cm

该藏由质地坚硬的黑色天然石料加工制成，外
呈八角形，内呈圆钵形，敞口，平底。通体磨光。
配棱柱形杵。制作精细，造型美观。

　　中华医学会 / 上海中医药大学医史博物馆藏

The collection is made of hard natural black stone.
It is octagon-shaped outside and bowl-shaped
inside. It has a flared mouth, a flat bottom, and a
polished body. A prismatic pestle goes with the
mortar. The artifact is delicately made and looks
artistic.

Preserved in Chinese Medical Association/ Museum
of Chinese Medicine, Shanghai University of
Traditional Chinese Medicine

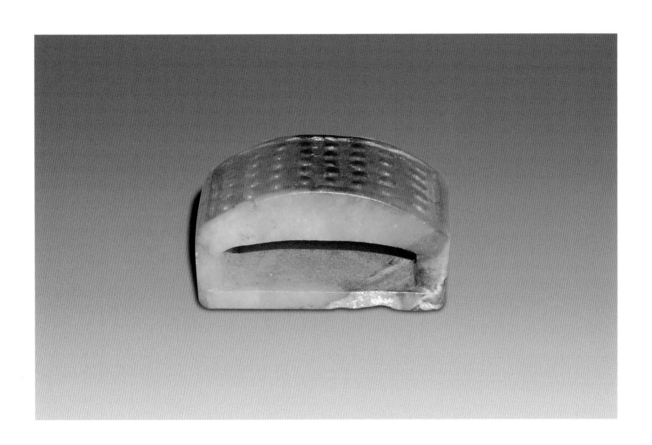

玉衣带扣

近现代

玉质

长 4 厘米，宽 2.8 厘米，高 2 厘米，重 100 克

Jade Buckle

Modern Times

Jade

Length 4 cm/ Width 2.8 cm/ Height 2 cm/ Weight 100 g

白色玉料雕琢而成。弓形，长方形底，弓面，

连珠纹。为生活器具。陕西省咸阳市秦都区

征集。

陕西医史博物馆藏

The buckle is made of white jade. It is shaped
like a bow with a triangular base and arced
surface decorated with pearl patterns. The
buckle was a common daily appliance. It was
collected in Qindu District of Xianyang City,
Shaanxi Province.

Preserved in Shaanxi Museum of Medical History

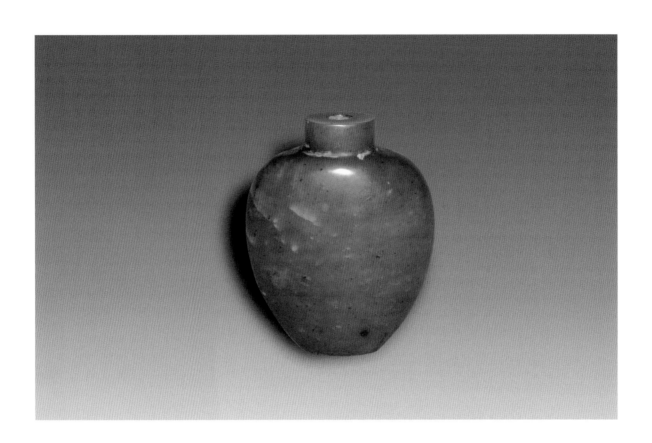

玉鼻烟壶

近现代

玉质

口径 1.8 厘米，底径 1.9 厘米，通高 6.1 厘米

Jade Snuff Bottle

Modern Times

Jade

Mouth Diameter 1.8 cm/ Bottom Diameter 1.9 cm/ Height 6.1 cm

完整碧玉雕琢而成。直口，扁腹，平底。用
于装鼻烟，为医药卫生器具。

陕西医史博物馆藏

The snuff bottle was carved out of green jade. It
has a straight mouth, an oblate belly, and a flat
bottom. The bottle was used for storing snuff
and it was used as a medical device.

Preserved in Shaanxi Museum of Medical History

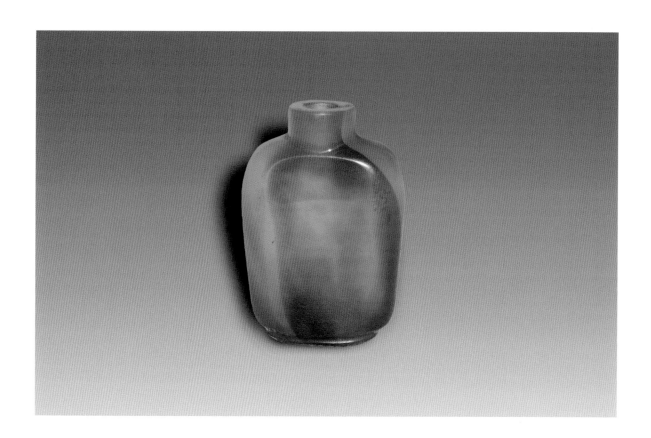

玉鼻烟壶

近现代

玉质

口径 1.5 厘米，底径 1.8 厘米，通高 5.4 厘米，重 53 克

Jade Snuff Bottle

Modern Times

Jade

Mouth Diameter 1.5 cm/ Bottom Diameter 1.8 cm/ Height 5.4 cm/ Weight 53 g

青玉雕琢而成。直口，扁腹，平底，中间镶
有一个红"寿"字。用于装鼻烟，为医药卫
生器具。

陕西医史博物馆藏

The bottle is made of green jade. It has a
straight mouth, an oblate belly, and a flat
bottom. The middle part is inlaid with a red
character "Shou" (longevity). The bottle was
used for storing snuff and it was used as a medical
device.

Preserved in Shaanxi Museum of Medical History

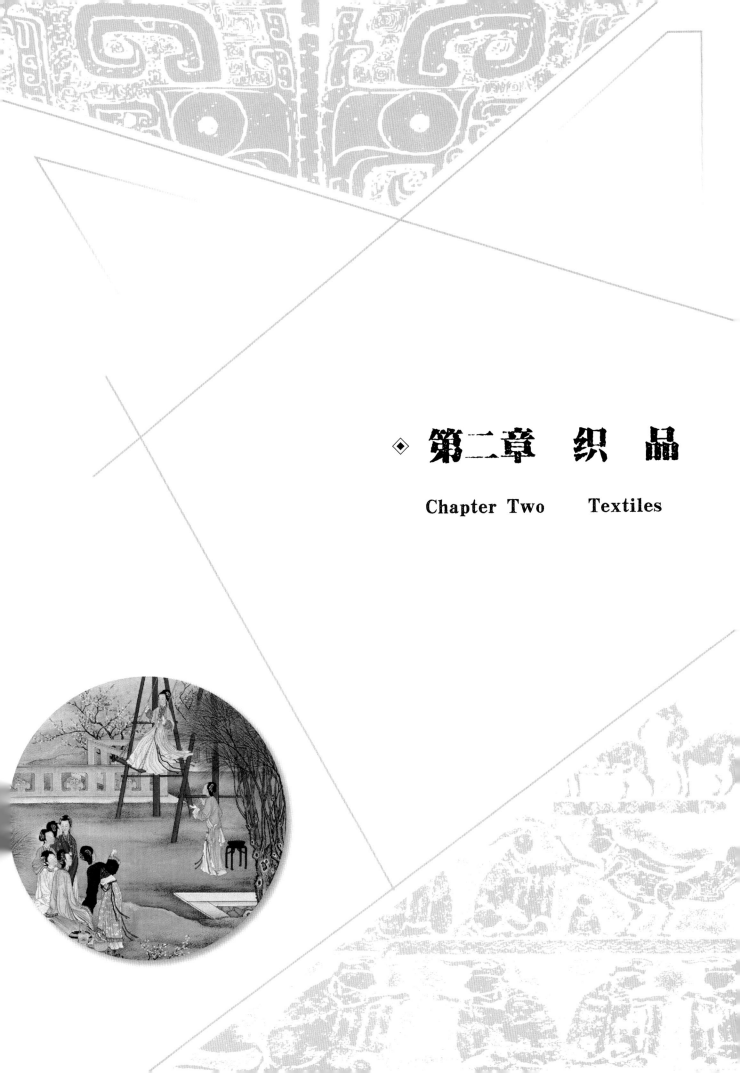

◇ 第二章 织 品

Chapter Two　　Textiles

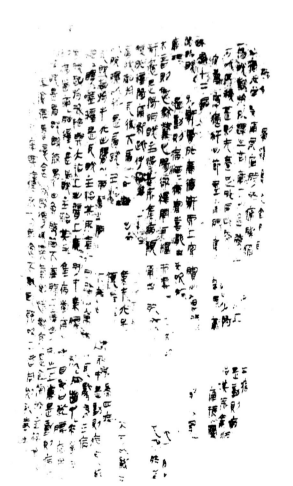

《阴阳十一脉灸经》（甲本）书影

西汉

丝质

长 30.5 厘米，宽 19.5 厘米

Printed Copy of *The Classic of Yin and Yang Eleven Meridians Acupuncture* (Form A)

Western Han Dynasty

Silk

Length 30.5 cm/ Width 19.5 cm

马王堆 3 号墓出土的 12 万字帛书中整理出来的《阴阳十一脉灸经》的书影，是迄今发现最早的、较全面记载了人体十一条经脉循行路线及所主疾病的著作，系我国发现最早的人体脉学和灸疗学专书之一。1973 年湖南省长沙市马王堆 3 号汉墓出土。

湖南省博物馆藏

The collection is a printed copy of *Yin Yang Shi Yi Mai Jiu Jing* (The Classic of Yin and Yang Eleven Meridians Acupuncture), which was sorted out of 120,000-word silk manuscripts excavated from Tomb No. 3 at Mawangdui. It is so far the earliest and relatively comprehensive book discovered that recorded eleven human body meridians and their main corresponding diseases. It is one of the earliest books on the sciences of the human body meridians and moxibustion in China. The artifact was excavated from Han Dynasty Tomb No. 3 at Mawangdui, Changsha City, Hunan Province, in 1973.

Preserved in Hunan Provincial Museum

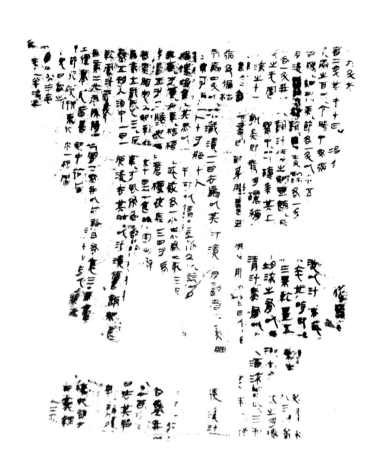

《养生方》书影

西汉

丝质

长 56 厘米，宽 31 厘米

Printed Copy of *Yang Sheng Fang*

Western Han Dynasty

Silk

Length 56 cm/ Width 31 cm

马王堆 3 号墓出土的 12 万字帛书中整理出来的《养生方》的书影。全书分四篇，即《十问》《合阴阳方》《杂禁方》《天下至道谈》，内容以养生、服食、吐纳、房中为主，而尤以"房中"为详细，是研究气功养生的可贵资料。1973 年湖南省长沙市马王堆 3 号汉墓出土。

湖南省博物馆藏

The collection is a printed copy of *Yang Sheng Fang* (Prescriptions for Health Maintenance) sorted out of 120,000-word silk manuscripts excavated from Han Dynasty Tomb No. 3 at Mawangdui. This book is divided into four sections, namely *Shi Wen* (the Ten Questions), *He Yin Yang Fang* (the Combination of Yin and Yang), *Za Jin Fang* (the Hybrid of Secret Recipes), and *Tian Xia Zhi Dao Tan* (Dao of the World). The main themes cover health maintenance, food therapy, inspiration and expiration, and sexual life, which is particularly detailed. The book is valuable for studying Qigong and health maintenance. It was excavated from Han Dynasty Tomb No. 3 at Mawangdui, Changsha City, Hunan Province, in 1973.
Preserved in Hunan Provincial Museum

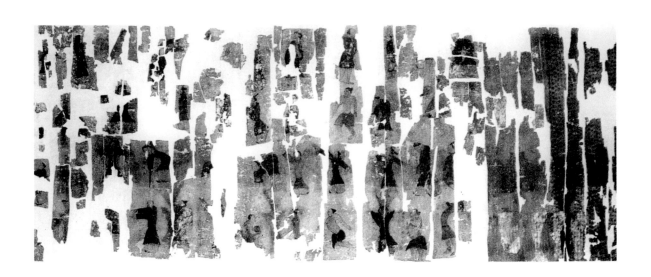

《导引图》帛画

西汉

丝质

长 133 厘米，宽 50 厘米

Silk Drawing of *Dao Yin Tu*

Western Han Dynasty

Silk

Length 133 cm/ Width 50 cm

这幅帛画共分四层，每层各有十一个在做各种导引动作的单人形象，男女共四十四人。图中的导引术式可以分为肢体运动、呼吸运动和器械运动三种类型。从每个导引术式旁所标注的文字来看，既有为治疗一定的疾病为主的术式，也有为健体御疾为主的术式，同时还有近一半是模仿野生动物动作的导引健体术式。此画是反映当时保健养生活动中导引术发展的重要内容。1973年湖南省长沙市马王堆3号西汉墓出土。

湖南省博物馆藏

Dao Yin Tu (Physical Exercises Chart), which was drawn on silk, is divided into four layers. On each layer there are eleven images of one person posing various physical exercise positions as a guidance. Men and women add up to forty-four. The positions in the chart fall into three types: limb movements, breathing exercises, and equipment-related movements. The words next to each guiding physical exercise position show that some positions aim not only at treating diseases and keeping fitness, but also building the body by imitating wild animals' movements. The chart reflects the contents of the development of breathing and physical exercises in health maintenance at that time. The artifact was excavated from Han Dynasty Tomb No. 3 at Mawangdui, Changsha City, Hunan Province, in 1973.

Preserved in Hunan Provincial Museum

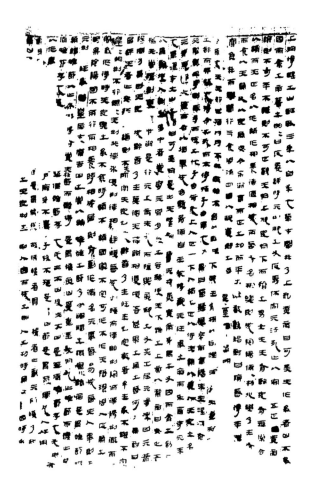

帛书《十大经·正乱》局部

西汉

丝质

高约 24 厘米

Part of Silk Book *Bringing Order to Turbulent Times*

Western Han Dynasty

Silk

Height 24 cm

此为专门记述黄帝战胜蚩尤之事的一篇帛书，其中有一段内容涉及了蹴鞠起源的传说：

"黄帝身禺〔遇〕之〔蚩〕尤，因而擒之……充其胃以为鞠，使人执之，多中者赏……"

作为蹴鞠起源之说，此虽为一神话传说，但反映出中国古代蹴鞠的起源是相当久远的。1973 年湖南省长沙市马王堆 3 号西汉墓出土。

湖南省博物馆藏

This article written on silk recorded the story that the Yellow Emperor defeated Chiyou, some of which involved the legends of the origin of cuju ball, the ancient football. Although the legend of the origin of cuju is a myth, it reflects that cuju ball of ancient Chinese people enjoys a very long history. The book was excavated from Han Dynasty Tomb No. 3 at Mawangdui, Changsha City, Hunan Province, in 1973. Preserved in Hunan Provincial Museum

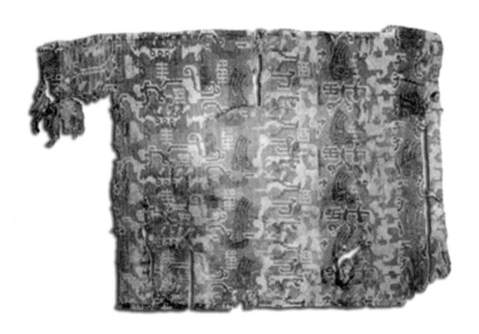

织锦（残片）

东汉

丝质

长 37.5 厘米，宽 24.5 厘米

Brocade (Fragments)

Eastern Han Dynasty

Silk

Length 37.5 cm/ Width 24.5 cm

锦以经线提花织成瑞兽纹，纹饰中可见隶书
"延年益寿，大宜子孙"字样。虽有残缺，
但瑞兽纹流畅并富有动感，图案色彩艳丽夺
目，表现了东汉时期织绣工艺的较高水平。
1980 年新疆罗布泊西岸楼兰古城东高台墓地
2 号墓出土。

新疆文物考古研究所藏

Auspicious animal patterns were woven with
jacquard on the brocade. Eight characters "Yan
Nian Yi Shou Da Yi Zi Sun", which mean
enjoying longevity and continuous prosperity of
the offspring, are written in official script in the
patterns. Although incomplete, the auspicious
animal patterns are smooth, vibrant and radiant,
which shows the high level of brocade making
in the Eastern Han Dynasty. The artifact was
excavated from Tomb No. 2 at the platform east
of the ancient city of Loulan, the west bank of
Luobupo, Xinjiang Autonomous Region, in
1980.

Preserved in Xinjiang Institute of Cultural
Relics and Archaeology

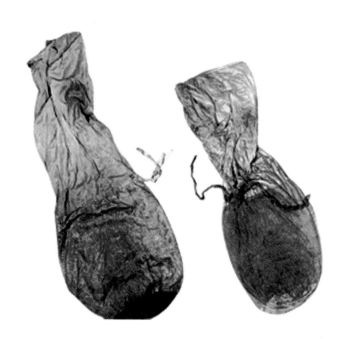

香囊

西汉

丝质

长 50 厘米，底径 13 厘米

Sachets

Western Han Dynasty

Silk

Length 50 cm/ Bottom Diameter 13 cm

左为信期绣囊，右为香色罗香囊。当时妇女随身佩带，取其芳香之气，或曰有避疫作用。1972 年湖南省长沙市马王堆 1 号汉墓出土。

湖南省博物馆藏

Sachets of the menstrual cycle and silk gauze are on the left and right respectively. Women in that period wore them for becoming fragrant or avoiding diseases. The sachets were excavated from Han Dynasty Tomb No. 1 at Mawangdui, Changsha City, Hunan Province, in 1972. Preserved in Hunan Provincial Museum

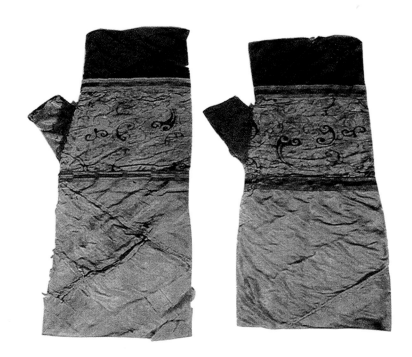

信期绣绢手套

西汉

丝质

长 24 厘米

Tough Silk Mittens of Menstrual Cycle

Western Han Dynasty

Silk

Length 24 cm

手套一双，无指套部分，五指裸露于外，便
于活动。表面饰卷云纹等彩色图案。1972 年
湖南省长沙市马王堆 1 号汉墓出土。

湖南省博物馆藏

The pair of mittens made it convenient for the
five fingers to move. It was decorated with
colored patterns of cirrus clouds. The artifact
was excavated from Han Dynasty Tomb No. 1
at Mawangdui, Changsha City, Hunan Province,
in 1972.

Preserved in Hunan Provincial Museum

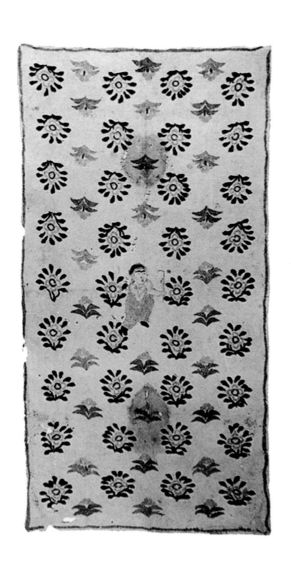

童子击球图花毡

唐

毛质

长 236 厘米

Colored Felt Patterned with a Ball-hitting Boy

Tang Dynasty

Fur

Length 236 cm

这是一件织造的花毡。花毡的图案由花朵和一名击球状的童子组成，击球的童子左手执一个弯月形球杖，正在弓身屈腿做击球状，在杖右方绘有一个球。整个图案生动地表现了唐代童子击球的场景。

日本正仓院藏

This is a colored woven felt with flower patterns and a boy hitting a ball. The child is holding a meniscus stick in his left hand and bending his back to hit the ball. There is a ball on the right side of the stick. The picture vividly shows the scene of a Tang Dynasty boy hitting the ball. Preserved in Shosoin, Japan

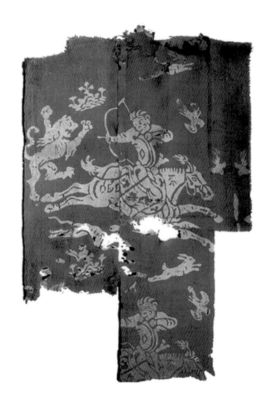

绛地射猎纹印花绢

唐

绢质

残长 43.5 厘米，宽 31.3 厘米

Tough Silk with Hand-printed Patterns of Hunting

Tang Dynasty

Silk

Residual Length 43.5 cm/ Width 31.3 cm

这件印花绢的纹饰，颇似一野外狩猎的真实场景。奔马上的骑士，注目回首，张弓满弦，正要射向张牙舞爪的猛狮。身上的弓袋、箭囊、宝剑、马鞍等具有装饰性的真实感。1972 年新疆维吾尔自治区吐鲁番县（今吐鲁番市）阿斯塔那 191 号墓出土。

吐鲁番博物馆藏

The pattern of the silk is like a real hunting scene. The rider with his head turning round is drawing the bow to shoot at a ferocious lion. The bow case, quiver, sword and saddle on the silk piece look almost real. The artifact was excavated from Tomb No. 191 in Asitana, Turfan County (now Turfan City), Xinjiang Autonomous Region, in. 1972. Preserved in Turfan Museum

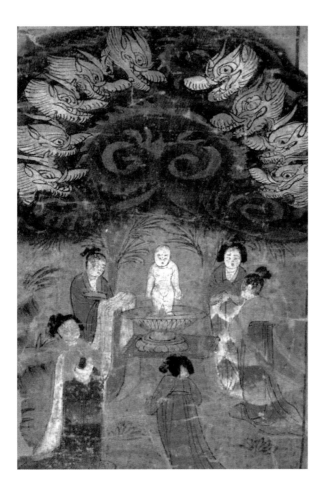

《九龙灌顶淋浴图》

唐

绢质

长 65.5 厘米，宽 19 厘米

Taking a shower with Nine Dragons Spraying Water from Above

Tang Dynasty

Silk

Length 65.5 cm/ Width 19 cm

为悉达太子淋浴图。太子站在俯莲座之仰莲盆内，九龙喷水淋浴太子，四周有宫女围立侍奉。敦煌莫高窟藏经洞出土。

大英博物馆藏

The artifact is a painting depicting Prince Xida taking a shower. The prince stands in an open lotus-shaped basin with a lotus-shaped base and nine dragons spray water over him. Maids standing beside serve him. Unearthed from the Library Cave of Dunhuang Mogao Grottoes. Preserved in British Museum

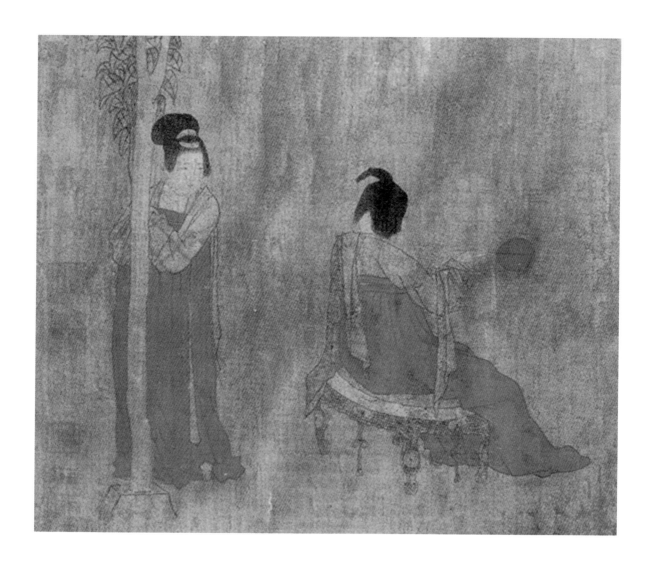

周昉《挥扇仕女图》卷局部

唐

绢质

原图：长 33.7 厘米，宽 204.8 厘米

该绢本描绘了宫廷妇女夏日纳凉、刺绣、理妆等生活情景。其中左侧一妇女倚树而立，右侧一妇女手持团扇背向而坐。

故宫博物院藏

Part of Silk Scroll of *Fanning Lady Drawing* by Zhou Fang

Tang Dynasty

Silk

Total Scroll: Length 33.7 cm/ Width 204.8 cm

The silk scroll depicts the palace women's daily life scenes such as enjoying cool air in summer, doing embroidery, and dressing up. One the left side a woman is standing against a tree and on the right side the other woman is sitting with her back facing the former while holding a moon-shaped fan in her hand.

Preserved in The Palace Museum

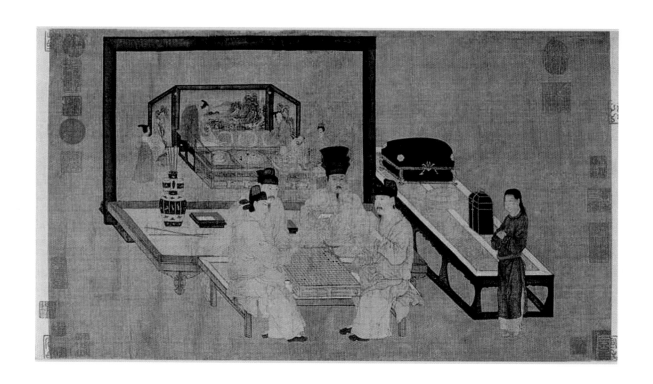

周文矩《重屏会棋图》卷

五代

绢质

长 40.3 厘米，宽 70.5 厘米

Silk Scroll of *Playing Chess Before Double Screens* Painted by Zhou Wenju

Five Dynasties

Silk

Length 40.3 cm/ Width 70.5 cm

此绢本描绘以南唐中主李璟为首的四人对坐下棋的情景。图中对弈的四人身后所置屏风上画有山水人物，并有一小屏风，因称"重屏会棋"。人物形象生动，用线细劲曲折，棋盘局面清晰，是一幅难得的反映五代时期弈棋内容的绘画作品。

故宫博物院藏

This silk scroll shows a scene that four people, led by Li Jing, the mid-major of the Southern Tang, are playing chess. The screen drawing with landscapes and figures behind the four people contain a small screen, so it is called "Chong Ping Hui Qi" (Playing Chess Before Double Screens). The figures were drawn vividly with fine and powerful lines. The situation of the chess game is clear too. It is a rare drawing which shows chess playing in the Five Dynasties.

Preserved in The Palace Museum

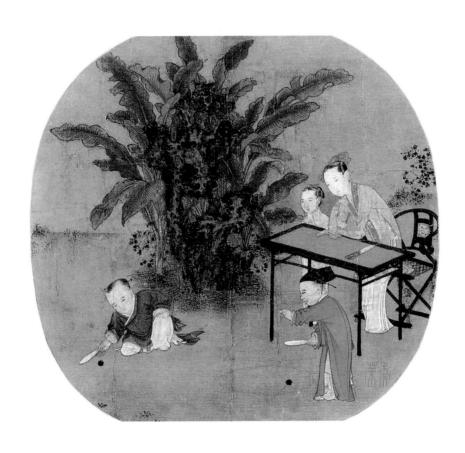

《蕉荫击球图》册页

宋

绢质

长 25 厘米，宽 24.5 厘米

Page of Drawing of *Hitting the Ball Under the Shade of a Musa Basjoo*

Song Dynasty

Silk

Length 25 cm/ Width 24.5 cm

图中两小儿各执一球板正在做击球游戏。画
面中配以芭蕉树和观赏石，使人物动作更显
活泼和具有真实性。

故宫博物院藏

The picture depicts two children playing a ball-
hitting game with a ball in each one's hand.
There are a Musa basjoo and ornamental stones
in the picture, which makes the figures and their
movements lively and realistic.
Preserved in The Palace Museum

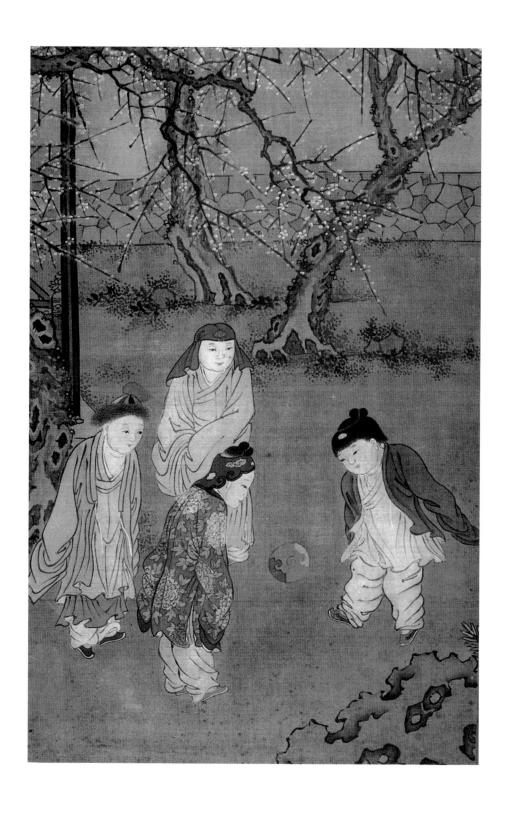

苏汉臣《长春百子图》卷局部

宋

绢质

原图：长 525.5 厘米，宽 30.6 厘米

这里选取的是百子图中童子蹴鞠的一个图案，图中四个童子围着一球在做蹴鞠游戏，画面清新，情趣浓厚。

故宫博物院藏

Part of Silk Scroll of *Hundred Children in Spring* Painted by Su Hanchen

Song Dynasty

Silk

Total Scroll: Length 525.5 cm/ Width 30.6 cm

This part is one of the pictures which depict a hundred boys playing. In the picture, four children are playing cuju ball as a game. The whole scene is fresh and interesting.

Preserved in The Palace Museum

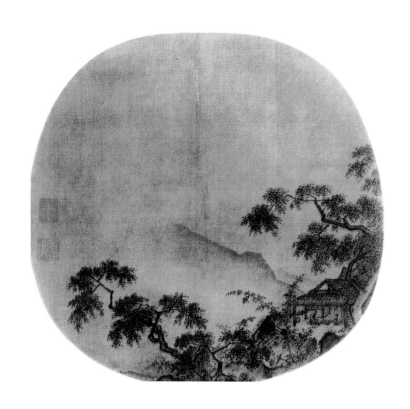

《山居对弈图》册页

宋

绢质

长 24.8 厘米，宽 24 厘米

Page of Painting of *Playing Chess in the Mountain*

Song Dynasty

Silk

Length 24.8 cm/ Width 24 cm

画面中隐约可见远处山势起伏，近景为茂盛的松树，山石、松林之间有一小屋，两位老者于屋内对坐而弈。图中山、树、山间小屋和棋者的布局，使整个画面更显静谧。

故宫博物院藏

There are undulating mountains, lush pine trees and rocks in the painting. Two old men are sitting in the small house among the objects and playing Chinese chess. The layout of the mountains, trees, house, and players makes the entire scene tranquil.

Preserved in The Palace Museum

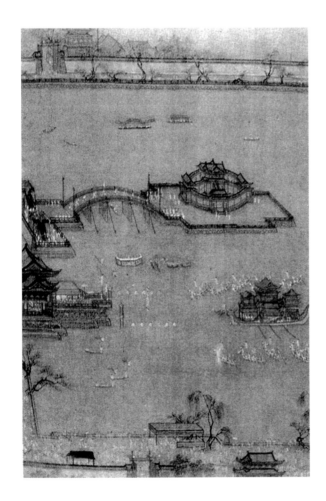

佚名《金明池争标图》局部

南宋

绢本，设色

纵 28.5 厘米，横 28.6 厘米

Part of *People Competing for the Post in Jinming Pool* by Anonymity

Southern Song Dynasty

Scroll, ink and colors on silk

Width 28.5 cm/ Length 28.6 cm

画面的中心是一巨型御用龙船，上承楼阁，宋帝正坐于楼中观看赛事。御船左、右各有五条龙舟，每舟十人，选手们正奋力划桨，奔向扎有锦旗的水上标竿。画面表现手法极为精细，颇具欢快气氛。图左下方用楷书署有"张择端进呈"五字，系后添款。

天津艺术博物馆

The center of the picture sits a giant imperial dragon boat connected to the Pavilion. Emperor of Song is sitting in the Pavilion to watch the competition. On each side of the imperial ship are five dragon boats respectively, and each boat has ten competitors. Those players are rowing their best to get the post with flag. The details of the picture are carefully designed and create a cheerful atmosphere. The five Chinese characters "Zhang Ze Duan Jin Cheng" on the left bottom were signed later in regular script. Preserved in Tianjin Art Museum

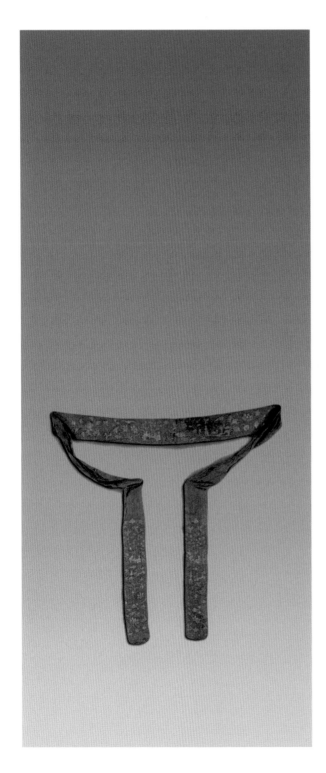

刺绣山水人物纹赭色绸裙带

元

丝质

长 155 厘米，宽 5 厘米

Dress Strap Embroidered with Patterns
of Landscape and Figures

Yuan Dynasty

Silk

Length 155 cm/ Width 5 cm

裙带长条状，由菱纹赭色绸缝制，束在女尸
夹裙之外。带中部及两端绣有纹饰，假山流
水，树木花草，持杖老翁凝视远方，幼童行
于小路，空中凤鸟祥云，一片园林景色，生
机盎然。1975 年邹城市李俨墓出土。

邹城市文物局藏

The long strap was sewn with hishimonoides
ochre silk and bundled outside the clip skirt
of a female corpse. The center and ends of
the strap were embroidered with patterns of
artificial hills, flowing water, trees and flowers,
an old man holding a stick and gazing into the
distance, a toddler walking on the path, flying
phoenixes and auspicious clouds in the air, all
of which form the lively scenery of a garden.
The artifact was excavated from Li Yan's tomb
in Zoucheng City, Shandong Province, in 1975.
Preserved in Zoucheng Municipal Bureau of
Cultural Relics

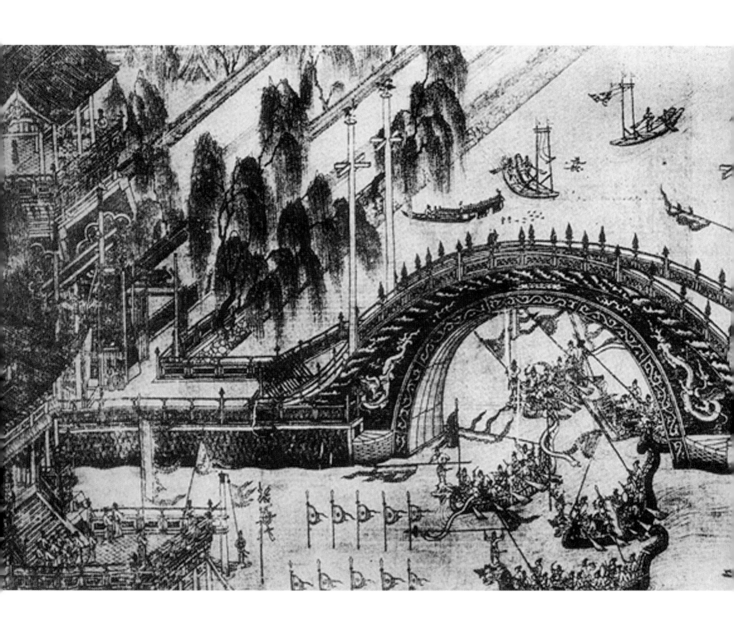

《龙舟夺标图·水秋千》卷局部

元

绢质

原画长 115 厘米，宽 25.1 厘米

这里选取的是画面中水手们做"水秋千"跳水表演的一个局部。高高的秋千，立于船的前部，跳水健儿从荡起的秋千板上飞身跃入水中。画面的描绘，生动真切，充满情趣，煞是精彩。

故宫博物院藏

Part of *Competing for Championship on Dragon Boats–Playing a Swing on Water*

Yuan Dynasty

Silk

Total Scroll: Length 115 cm/ Width 25.1 cm

This is a part of the picture which depicts the seamen performing a swing on water. The high swing is placed in the front of a boat and the seamen jump into the water from the highly-swaying swing. The picture is full of fun and excitement.

Preserved in The Palace Museum

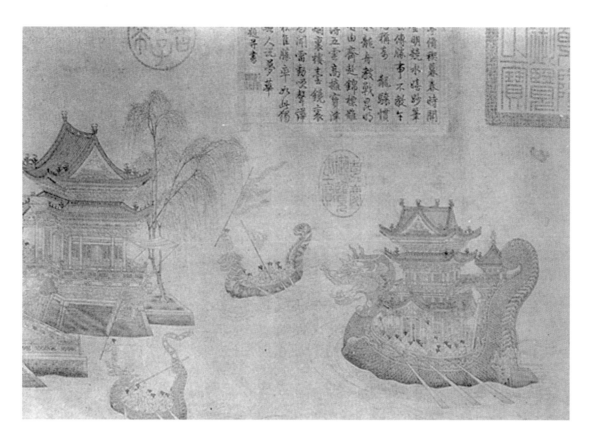

王振鹏《龙池竞渡图》局部

元

绢质

原图：长 243.8 厘米，宽 30.2 厘米

Part of Boat Race in Dragon Pool **Painted by Wang Zhenpeng**

Yuan Dynasty

Silk

Total Scroll: Length 243.8 cm/ Width 30.2 cm

这是画家根据北宋崇宁年间（1102—1106）三月三日由皇家在金明池举办的龙舟竞渡之盛况绘制而成的。画面对当时龙舟夺标的赛况进行了形象的描绘，整体白描，不设色。

台北故宫博物院藏

The artist painted the frame based on the grand scene that the royalties held a dragon boat race at Jinming Pool on the third of the third lunar month during Chongning Period (1102–1106) of the North Song Dynasty. The picture depicts the vivid scene of competing for the dragon boat championship. The picture was painted with line drawing without colors.

Preserved in National Palace Museum

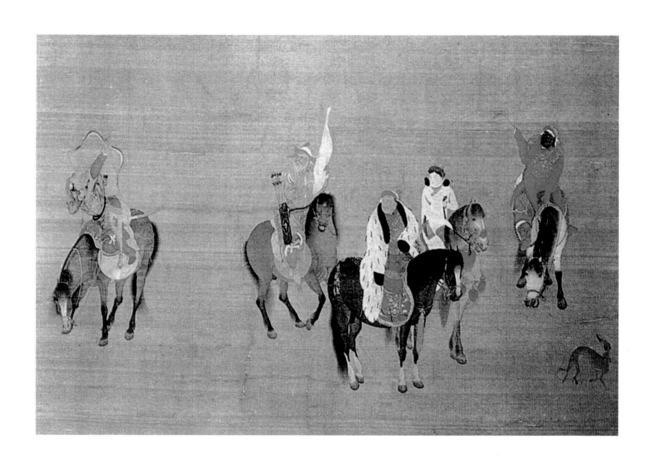

刘贯道《元世祖射猎图》局部

元

绢本，设色

原图：纵 182.9 厘米，横 104.1 厘米

Part of *Hunting Painting of Khubilai Khan, Shizu of Yuan* by Liu Guandao

Yuan Dynasty

Scroll, ink and colors on silk

Total Scroll: Width 182.9 cm/ Length 104.1 cm

此图描绘了元世祖忽必烈（1260—1294 年在位）率领百官在郊野骑马执弓射猎的情景。

台北故宫博物院藏

The painting is one with tinted color. The painting shows Khubilai Khan (reigned from 1260–1294), Shizu of Yuan, and his officials are riding on horses and hunting with bows and arrows in the suburbs.

Preserved in National Palace Museum

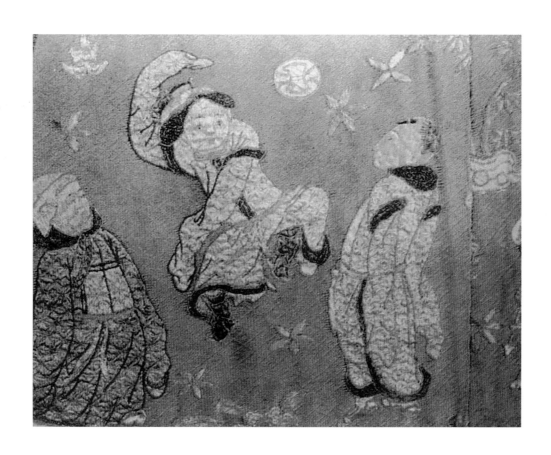

女夹衣《百子戏图》局部

明

丝质

原件夹身长 71 厘米，通袖长 163 厘米，下摆宽 81.5 厘米

Part of Picture with Patterns of *A Hundred Playing Children* in Female Lined Dress

Ming Dynasty

Silk

Length of Original Lined Dress 71 cm/ Sleeve Length 163 cm/ Bottom Width 81.5 cm

这件夹衣为明孝靖皇后之物，图案均绣于胸及两袖上。在夹衣所绣蹴鞠图案中，有三个少年在做蹴鞠游戏，中间一人正腾身以足踢球，两边的伙伴在聚精会神地盯着被踢起的皮球，画面生动有趣。1956—1958 年北京市昌平县（今昌平区）明定陵出土。

定陵博物馆藏

This piece of clothes belonged to Queen Xiaojing of the Ming Dynasty. All the patterns are embroidered on the chest and both sleeves. In the cuju ball-playing picture, three teenagers are playing the ball. One of them is jumping to kick the ball and the other two teenagers are looking attentively at the ball. The whole scene is very vivid and interesting. This artifact was excavated from Dingling Mausoleum of the Ming Dynasty in Changping County (now Changping District), Beijing, between 1956 and 1958.

Preserved in Dingling Museum

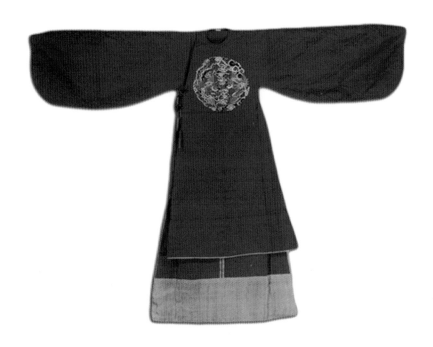

绣双凤补赭红缎长袍

明

丝质

前身长 113 厘米，后身长 147 厘米，通袖长 306 厘米，袖口宽 13 厘米

Auburn Satin Robe Embroidered with Double Phoenixes

Ming Dynasty

Silk

Front Length 113 cm/ Back Length 147 cm/ Sleeve Length 306 cm/ Sleeve Width 13 cm

为曲阜市孔府旧藏。暗花赭红缎，盘领，右衽，瘦长，后身长于前身，两袖宽肥，袖口狭小。胸背缀有凤补，五彩丝线绣出双凤，舞于祥云之中。此袍系明代衍圣公夫人礼服，随衍圣公一品官服由皇帝赐予。

山东博物馆藏

This long and narrow robe, which was originally collected in Duke Yansheng Mansion, Qufu City, is made of auburn satin with dark flowery patterns. Its collar is coiled, the right front flap covers the left one, and its back side is longer than the front one. It has two broad sleeves but narrow cuffs. On its upper mid-front and back are double phoenixes embroidered with colorful silk threads, which dance among auspicious cloud patterns. This robe, a formal dress of the wife of Duke Yansheng of the Ming Dynasty, was bestowed by the emperor along with Duke Yansheng's first-rank official costume.

Preserved in Shandong Museum

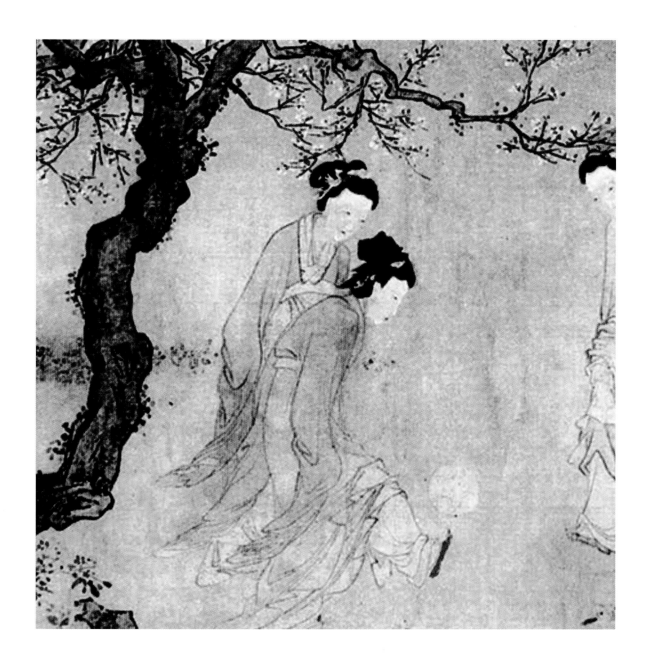

杜堇《仕女图》卷局部

明

绢质

纵 30.5 厘米，横 168.9 厘米

《仕女图》卷是以描绘唐代宫廷妇女生活为内容的长卷，全卷共八段。本图选取的是其中"蹴鞠"的一段画面。描绘了三名女子于树下蹴鞠的场景，人物形象生动细腻。

上海博物馆藏

Part of Silk Scroll of *Beautiful Ladies* Painted by Du Jin

Ming Dynasty

Silk

Width 30.5 cm/ Length 168.9 cm

The picture depicts the palace women's daily life in the Tang Dynasty. The whole picture is divided into eight parts. This part is the scene of three women playing the cuju ball under a tree. The figures were painted vividly and exquisitely.

Preserved in Shanghai Museum

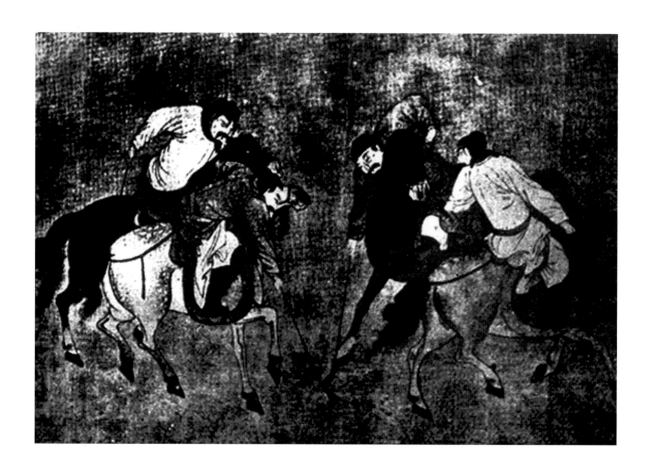

明人临摹《宋人击球图》

明

绢质

纵 47 厘米，横 43.2 厘米

Imitated Picture of *Song Dynasty People Hitting the Ball*

Ming Dynasty

Silk

Length 47 cm/ Width 43.2 cm

图中四位击球者头戴折角巾，身着长袍，均
为宋人装束。他们骑在马上挥舞球杖正在奋
力击球。画面将四人策马击球的激烈状态刻
画得细致入微，极为生动。

英国维多利亚和阿尔伯特博物馆藏

The four players in the picture are wearing
robes in the style of the Song Dynasty. They are
riding horses and struggling to hit the ball. The
picture depicts vividly the tense scene of the
four people on horseback hitting the ball.

Preserved in Victoria and Albert Museum, London

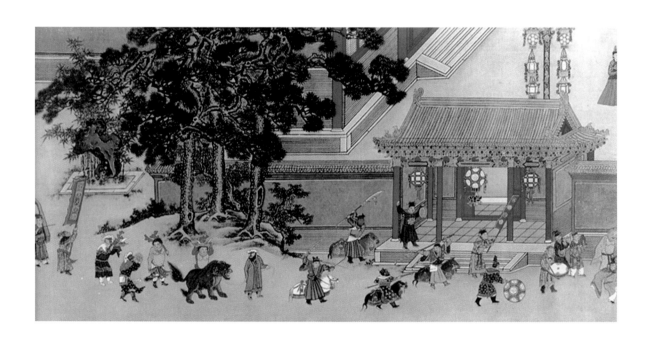

《明宪宗元宵行乐图卷》局部

明

绢本，设色

原图：纵 37 厘米，横 624 厘米

Partial Painting of *the Grand Occasion on Lantern Festival during the Period of Xianzong of Ming*

Ming Dynasty

Scroll, ink and colors on silk

Total Scoll: Width 37 cm/ Length 624 cm

该图描绘的是明代元宵节（农历正月十五日）宫中行乐的盛况。这里选取的是其中的一个局部画面，武士们分别执剑、枪和刀等器械在做各种武艺对练和单练的表演。此当为元宵节娱乐的内容之一。

中国国家博物馆藏

The whole scroll depicts the grand occasion in the court in the lantern festival during the Ming period. This scene shows that warriors holding swords, spears and blades perform all kinds of martial arts, which is one of the entertainments in the lantern festival.

Preserved in National Museum of China

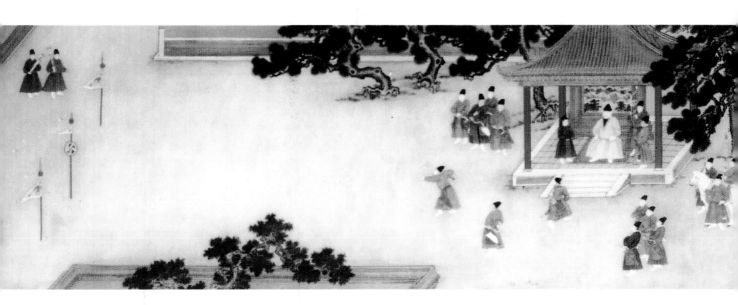

《明宣宗行乐图》卷局部

明

绢质

原图：纵 36.8 厘米，横 688.5 厘米

Part of Picture of *Xuanzong's Pleasure Seeking*

Ming Dynasty

Silk

Total Scoll: Length 36.8 cm/ Width 688.5 cm

这是一幅以明宣宗朱瞻基于宫中行乐为主题
绘制的画卷，此为其中一段。画面中，明宣
宗正于亭内观看大臣们射箭比武，这是明代
宫中射箭活动的真实描绘。

故宫博物院藏

This is a silk scroll of Ming Emperor Zhu
Zhanji seeking pleasure in the palace. And
this is one part of it. In the picture, the Ming
emperor is watching the ministers taking an
archery contest. This picture depicts true to life
archery contests held in the palace in the Ming
Dynasty.

Preserved in The Palace Museum

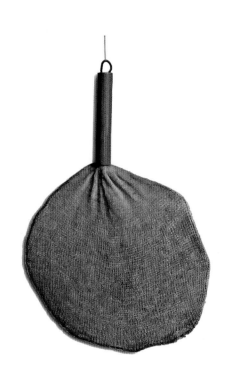

药物过滤网

清

竹、棉纱、铁质

长 15.6 厘米，宽 10.5 厘米

Medicine Filter

Qing Dynasty

Bamboo, cotton yarn and iron

Length 15.6 cm/ Width 10.5 cm

该藏由竹柄、棉纱网、铁丝圈构成。柄部书"春生堂"字样。为过滤药物的器具。

中华医学会 / 上海中医药大学医史博物馆藏

The collection consists of a bamboo handle, a cotton yarn net, and an iron wire ring, The handle is inscribed with the name of the drugstore "Chun Sheng Tang". The artifact was used for filtering drugs.

Preserved in Chinese Medical Association/ Museum of Chinese Medicine, Shanghai University of Traditional Chinese Medicine

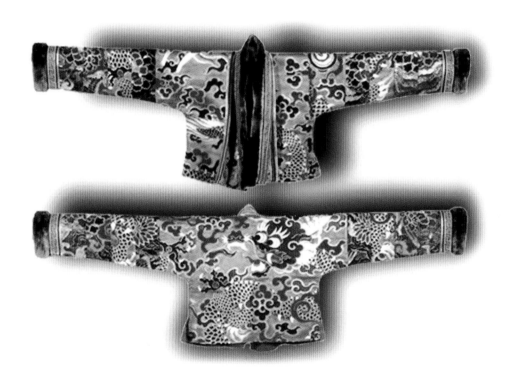

龙纹短上衣

17—19 世纪

缎，锦绣

长 192 厘米，宽 58 厘米

Short Upper Outer Garment with Dragon Patterns

17th to 19th Century

Satin

Length 192 cm/ Width 58 cm

黄缎，锦绣，长袖对襟，身长至腰。绣一条龙盘旋回绕于衣袖间，龙首位于后身右上，龙尾止于右前襟。应为皇帝所赐衣物。

西藏博物馆藏

The yellow satin upper garment, with buttons down the front, is short but has long sleeves. A coiling dragon is embroidered on the body and sleeves, with its head on the back of the upper right side and its tail on the right front piece. The garment was supposed to be granted by an emperor.

Preserved in Tibet Museum

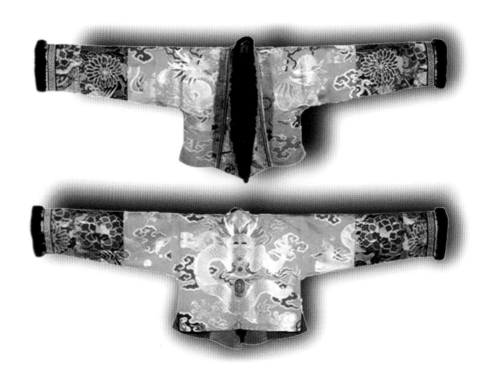

龙纹短上衣

17—19 世纪

缎，锦绣

长 194 厘米，宽 58 厘米

Short Upper Outer Garment with Dragon Patterns

17th to 19th Century

Satin

Length 194 cm/ Width 58 cm

黄缎，锦绣，长袖对襟，身长至腰。左、右
前襟各绣一龙，龙首相向而对。上衣后身绣
一条龙盘旋。为皇帝所赐衣物。

西藏博物馆藏

The yellow satin upper garment, with buttons
down the front, is short but has long sleeves.
On both sides of the front part are embroidered
two dragons with their heads facing each other.
The rear of the upper garment is embroidered
with a coiling dragon pattern. The garment was
granted by an emperor.

Preserved in Tibet Museum

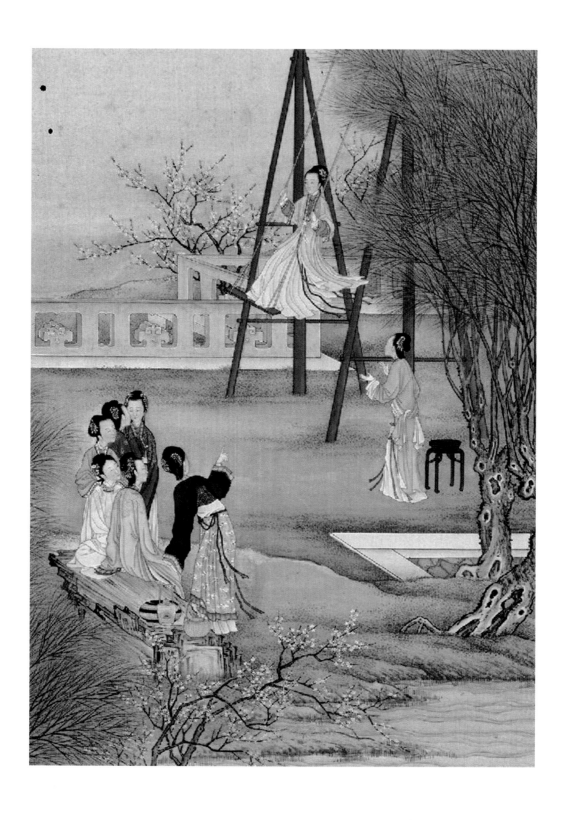

陈枚《月曼清游图册·秋千图》

清

绢质

长 37 厘米，宽 31.8 厘米

《月曼清游图册》设色绢本共 12 幅，描写宫廷仕女十二个月寻梅、赏花、吟诗玩月的深闺享乐生活。本图为其中一幅，画老柳吐芽，桃花盛开之际，曲栏旁一仕女在荡秋千，旁边仕女或坐或立观赏景色，以享春光之乐。人物形态生动，富于初春气息。

故宫博物院藏

Part of *Pleasure Seeking Album–Swing* Painted by Chen Mei

Qing Dynasty

Silk

Length 37 cm/ Width 31.8 cm

Yue Man Qing You Tu Ce (Pleasure Seeking Album) consists of 12 silk pictures which describe court ladies' pleasure-seeking life in the palace during the 12 months of the year. In this picture an old willow tree is sprouting and peach trees are blooming. Beside the railing, a court lady is playing on a swing while the others sitting or standing are enjoying the splendor of early spring. The characters in the picture are depicted lively.

Preserved in The Palace Museum

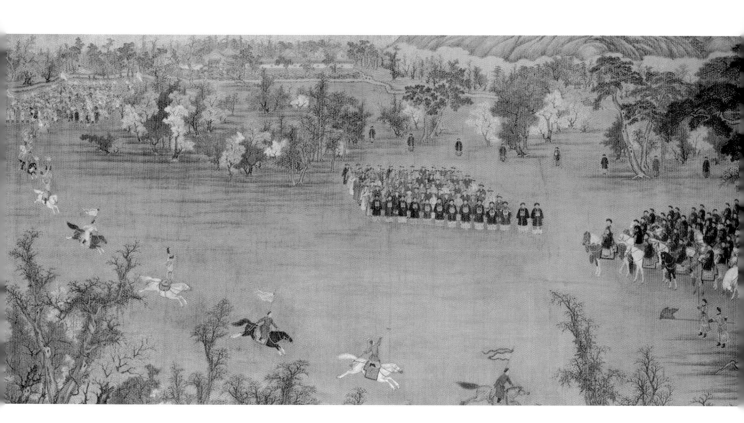

郎世宁等《马术图》局部

清

绢质

原画：长 426.2 厘米，宽 223.4 厘米

Part of *Horsemanship* Painted by Lang Shining

Qing Dynasty

Silk

Total Scroll: Length 426.2 cm/ Width 223.4 cm

画面是以清乾隆皇帝在文武百官和归附的土尔扈特首领们陪同下，于承德避暑山庄观看马术表演为背景绘制的。图中，骑士们由画面左上方集结地点出发，鱼贯驰过皇帝及其大臣面前，并在马上表演着各种技巧动作。全图布局宏伟，气氛热烈，极具运动感。

故宫博物院藏

The picture describes the scene that with the company of hundreds of his officials and chiefs of submitted Torghut tribe, Emperor Qianlong is watching a horseback riding in Chengde Summer Resort. The riders setting out together at the upper left side of the picture. They pass in front of the emperor and the ministers in succession, making various stunting movements on horseback. The layout of this picture is magnificent and the exciting atmosphere makes the scene full of vitality.

Preserved in The Palace Museum

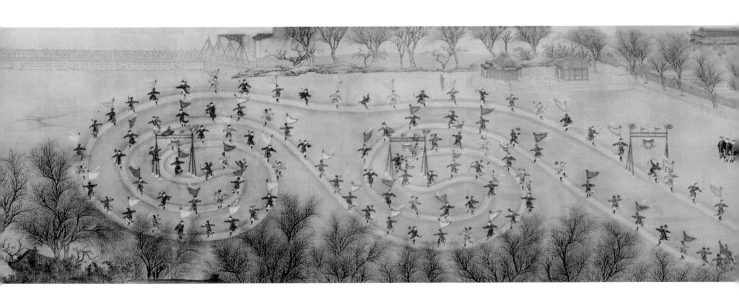

金昆、程至道、福隆安《冰嬉图》卷局部

清

绢质

原图：长 578.8 厘米，宽 35 厘米

Part of *Performances on Ice* Painted by Jin Kun, Cheng Zhidao, and Fu Long'an

Qing Dynasty

Silk

Total Scroll: length 578.8 cm/ Width 35 cm

这幅长卷以清代的中海为背景，对当时宫廷冰嬉表演的壮观场面及种种细节都做了相当真实、具体的描绘。其中既有冰上花样和杂技的表演，又有如同今天的速度滑冰的形式，反映出滑冰这一运动项目在清代已经具有相当高的水平了。

故宫博物院藏

This long picture makes a realistic and vivid depiction of the magnificent scene of court ice performances in the Qing Dynasty with the Central Lake as the background. The figure skating and acrobatics on the ice in the picture are similar to today's speed skating. It reflects that skating reached a high level as a sport in the Qing Dynasty.

Preserved in The Palace Museum

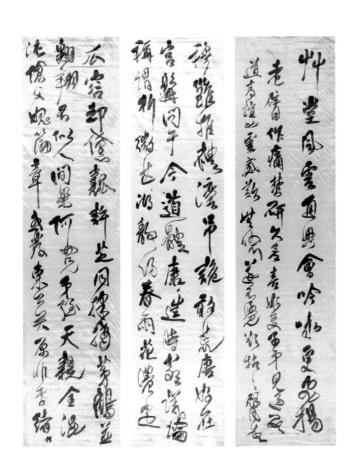

傅山草书《寿王锡予四十二韵》十二条屏（部分）

清

绫本

纵 200 厘米，横 51.1 厘米

Poem Screen of Fu Shan's Cursive Script (partial)

Qing Dynasty

Silk

Length 200 cm/ Width 51.1 cm

草书写五言四十韵诗，题鉴"五福堂珍藏"，钤"傅山印""五福堂"印。十二屏钤有"黄绍斋家珍藏"印及"少斋六十后所得"印。

山西博物院藏

On the screen, a poem with five characters to a line and 40 rhymes is written in cursive script, with the inscriptions meaning "preserved in Wufutang" and two seals of Fu Shan and Wufutang. On the 12th screen there are also two seals meaning "preserved by Huang Shaozhai" and so on.

Preserved in Shanxi Museum

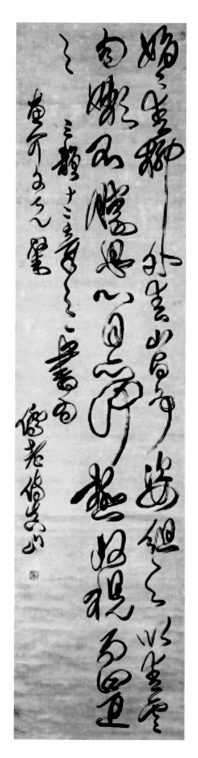

傅山草书《五律诗》轴

清

绫本

纵 202 厘米，横 51 厘米

墨迹，草书。书行笔迅疾如飞，流利酣畅，气势雄浑，有龙蛇飞舞之势。

故宫博物院藏

Calligraphy Scroll of Poem by Fu Shan

Qing Dynasty

Silk

Length 202 cm/ Width 51 cm

This calligraphy work is a cursive script with ink on the silk. The brush strokes are smooth and swift, which presents a magnificent and vigorous style.

Preserved in The Palace Museum

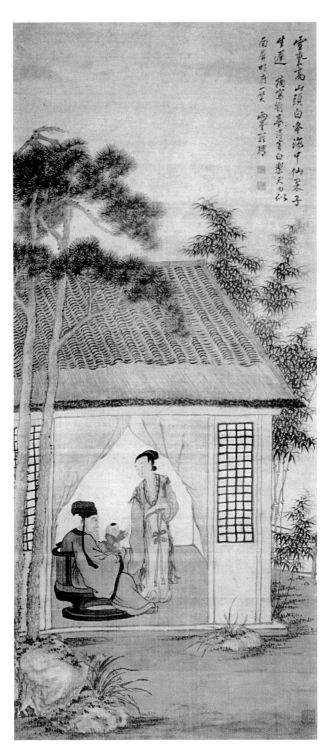

罗聘《得子图》轴

清

绢本

纵 107.5 厘米，横 47.5 厘米

山西博物院藏

Luo Pin's Painting Scroll of *Siring a Child*

Qing Dynasty

Silk

Length 107.5 cm/ Width 47.5 cm

Preserved in Shanxi Museum

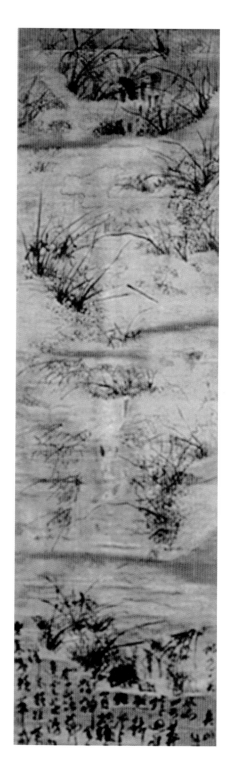

傅山《云兰图》轴

清

绫本

纵 108 厘米，横 52.5 厘米

Fu Shan's Painting Scroll of Cloud and Orchid

Qing Dynasty

Silk

Length 108 cm/ Width 52.5 cm

画中兰草漫山遍野，连云带水，用笔简洁，构
图新颖，自题五言诗一首："老来无赖笔，瀰
沢太滇狂，带水连云出，漫山驾岭薇。精神全
不肖，色取似非常，三盏醮新榨，回头笑莽苍。"
款署"枫兄一笑，真山"，钤"傅山印"。

山西博物院藏

This painting depicts the scene of rampant
orchids, floating clouds and flowing water. The
whole painting is concisely sketched with novel
and unique layout. There is also a five-character
octave of the painter, as well as the signature and
the signet stamp.

Preserved in Shanxi Museum

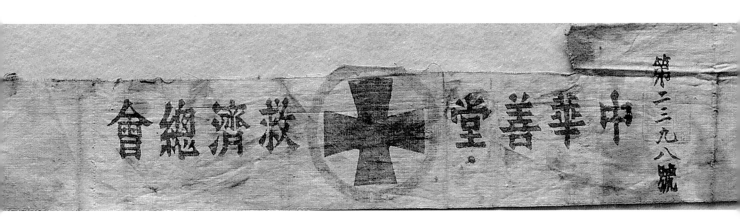

蓝十字总会袖标

民国时期

土布

长 40 厘米，宽 10 厘米

Armband for Blue Cross Charitable Institution

Republican Period

Home-made cloth

Length 40 cm/ Width 10 cm

为抗战期间蓝十字总会袖标，狭长的横长方形，中心为红圈蓝十字图案，两侧分别横书"中华善堂""救济总会"，最右侧小号字体竖书"第二三九八号"。蓝十字总会亦称新加坡中华善堂救济总会，成立于 20 世纪 40 年代。该总会及其属下各善堂，专注于救济灾难、扶助贫困等慈善公益事业。

上海医药文献博物馆藏

The armband used by Blue Cross Charitable Institution during the War of Resistance Against Japanese Aggression is a narrow and long horizontal rectangle with a blue cross in a red circle in the center. On the two sides are written horizontally four words separately, meaning Chinese Charitable Institution and Charitable Institution, respectively. On the very right side is written vertically small characters "No. 2398". Blue Cross Charitable Institution, also known as Singapore Tiong Hwa Siang Tin Kieu Chi Chong Hua, was founded in the 1940s. It and its branches were devoted to charities causes like helping people in disasters and poverty.

Preserved in Shanghai Medical Literature Museum

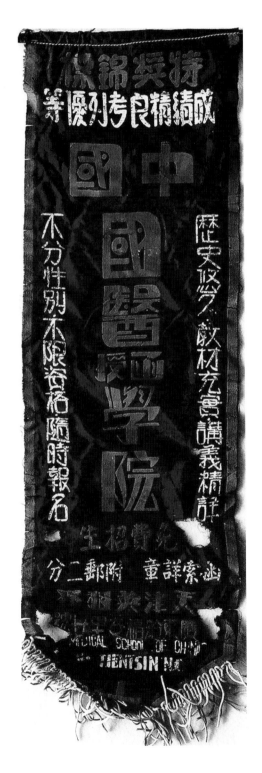

锦旗

民国时期

丝绸

长 60 厘米，宽 10 厘米

Silk Banner

Republican Period

Silk

Length 60 cm/ Width 10 cm

狭长的纵长方形，蓝底红边，最上部有红字横书，字体残缺，其下白字横书"成绩精良考列优等"，其下红字横书"中国"，其下红字纵书"国医函授学院"，其两侧白字分别纵书"历史悠久 教材充实 讲义精辟""不分性别 不限资格 随时报名"，再往下红、白色字体依次横书，除"免费招生"外，其余已模糊难辨。系1938年天津中国国医函授学院特奖锦标，可作奖赏和广告宣传用。

上海医药文献博物馆藏

The silk banner is a narrow and long vertical rectangle with a blue background and red rims. On its very top are broken red characters. At its bottom are horizontally written eight white words meaning ranking first class for excellent grades, under which are red horizontal words meaning China and red vertical words meaning Correspondence School of Traditional Chinese Medicine. On its both sides are vertically white words separately meaning long history, rich-content textbook and penetrating teaching materials; and register at any time without constraint of gender or qualification. Under them are horizontal red and white words in turn. All the words except four ones meaning free enrollment are too vague to be recognized. This banner was used by Tianjin Correspondence School of Traditional Chinese Medicine in 1938 as a grand prize. It could be used as an award or for publicity.

Preserved by Shanghai Medical Literature Museum

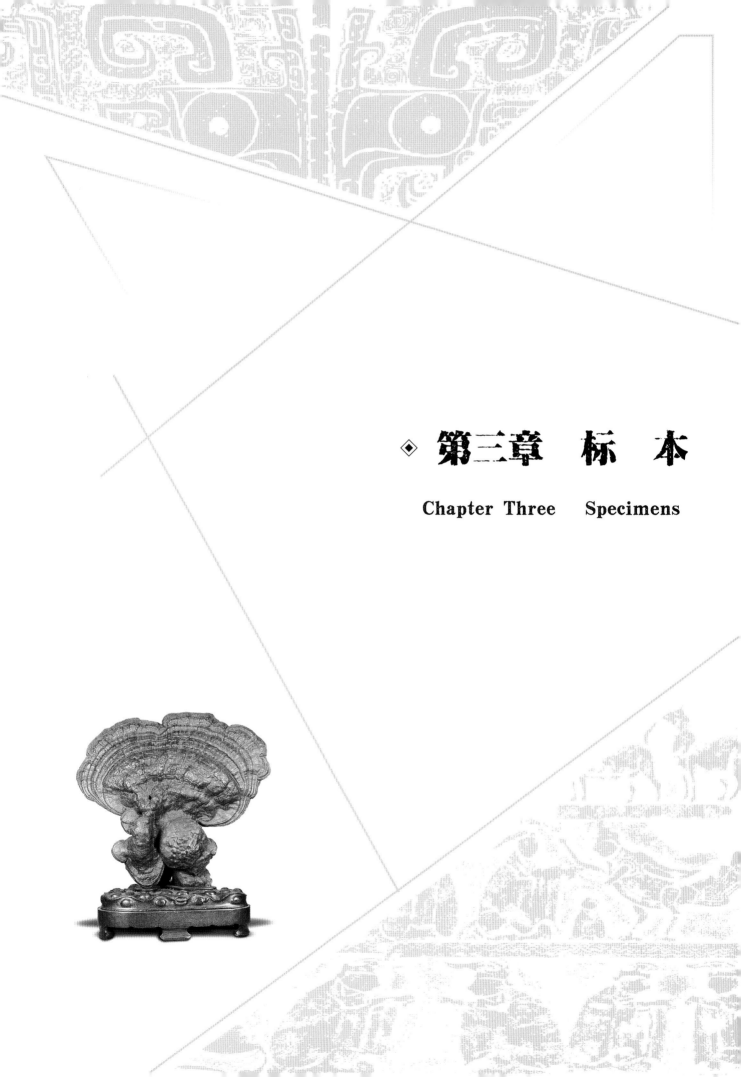

◈ 第三章 标 本

Chapter Three   Specimens

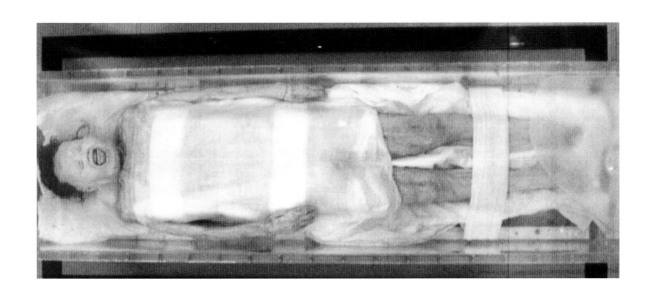

西汉女尸

西汉

古尸

身长 1.54 米，体重 34.3 千克

Female Corpse of the Western Han Dynasty

Western Han Dynasty

Ancient corpse

Height 1.54 m/ Weight 34.3 kg

系西汉长沙国丞相轪候利苍的妻子，名辛追。尸体出土时扎有九道丝带，裹衣衾 20 层。皮肤呈浅黄褐色，润泽而有弹性。外形与内脏器官均完整。经病理解剖查明，死于胆绞痛诱发冠心病致猝死，时年 50 岁左右。1972 年湖南省长沙市马王堆 1 号汉墓出土。

湖南省博物馆藏

She, Xin Zhui, was the wife of Li Cang, who was the prime minister of Changsha in the Western Han Dynasty. The body was tied with nine bundles of silk ribbons and wrapped with twenty layers of clothes and quilt when it was excavated. The skin of the body is tawny, glossy and elastic. The skin and internal organs are intact. Autopsy verified that she died of coronary heart disease due to cholecystalgia when she was 50 years old. The corpse was excavated from Han Dynasty Tomb No. 1 at Mawangdui, Changsha City, Hunan Province, in 1972.

Preserved in Hunan Provincial Museum

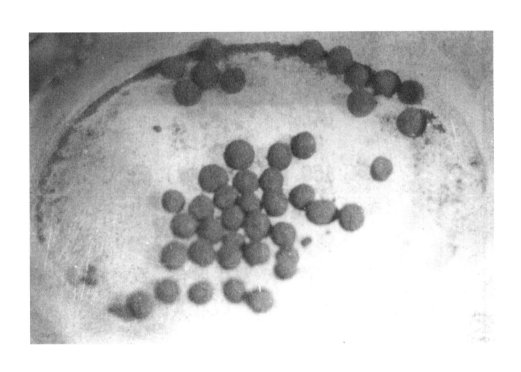

丹丸

东晋

化合物

直径 0.5 厘米

Pills

Eastern Jin Dynasty

Chemical compound

Diameter 0.5 cm

丹丸 100 余粒，粉红色，呈颗粒状，为古代
道家、神仙家炼制的丹药。据传服食可以升仙，
也可作药用。1965 年在南京北郊象山 7 号墓
（东晋升平三年王丹虎墓）出土，出土时安
放在一漆盘内（盘已朽）。

上海中医药博物馆藏

The collection includes about 100 grains of pink
pills, which were the medicine ancient Taoists
made. It is said that the pills could make people
become immortal beings after they took them
and could also be used as medicine. The pills
were put in a lacquered tray (which is rotten)
when it was excavated from Tomb No. 7 of the
third year of Shengpin Period of the Eastern Jin
Dynasty at Elephant Mountain, Nanjing City, in
1965.
Preserved in Shanghai Museum of Traditional
Chinese Medicine

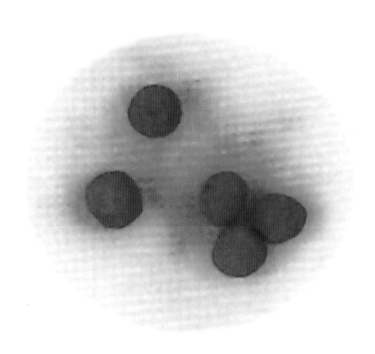

丹丸

东晋

化合物

直径 0.4 ~ 0.6 厘米

Pills

Eastern Jin Dynasty

Chemical compound

Diameter 0.4−0.6 cm

丹丸 5 粒，红色，呈颗粒状，表面有轻度风化。
为古代道家、神仙家炼制的丹药。据传服食可
以升仙，也可作药用。1965 年南京王丹虎墓
出土。南京市博物馆调拨，1973 年入藏。

中华医学会 / 上海中医药大学医史博物馆藏

The collection includes five grains of slightly
weathered red pills, which were the medicine
that ancient Taoists made. It is said that the pills
could make people become immortal beings after
they took them and could also be used as medicine.
The pills were excavated from Wang Danhu's tomb
in Nanjing in 1965 and were allocate by Nanjing
Municipal Museum in 1973.
Preserved in Chinese Medical Association/ Museum
of Chinese Medicine, Shanghai University of
Traditional Chinese Medicine

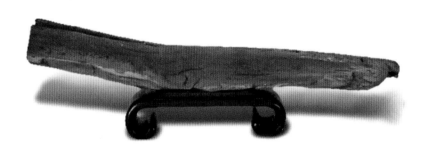

香料

宋

木质

长 27 厘米，宽 4.6 厘米

Spice

Song Dynasty

Wood

Length 27 cm/ Width 4.6 cm

段枝状，表面有轻度风化。为古代香料之一，用东南亚所产檀香木枝干制成。这批香料来源于 1973 年 8 月在福建泉州湾后渚港发掘出土的一艘宋代海船中。宋代时任泉州市舶司提举的赵汝适在《诸蕃志》中记录了当时中外商贸交易的一些情况。

中华医学会 / 上海中医药大学医史博物馆藏

The spice is shaped like a tree branch and its surface is slightly weathered. As one type of the ancient spices in Southeast Asia, it is made of sandalwood branches. The spice came from a Song Dynasty ship which was excavated in Houzhu Port, Quanzhou Bay, Fujian Province, in August 1973. Zhao Rushi, who was the trade administration official of Quanzhou City at that time in the Song Dynasty, recorded the trade between China and foreign countries in *Zhu Pan Zhi* (A Collection of Geography of Various Countries).
Preserved in Chinese Medical Association/ Museum of Chinese Medicine, Shanghai University of Traditional Chinese Medicine

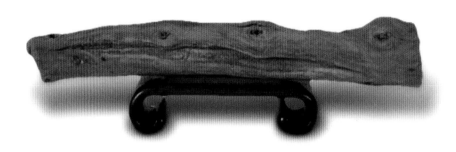

香料

宋

木质

长 24.5 厘米，宽 3.8 厘米

Spice

Song Dynasty

Wood

Length 24.5 cm/ Width 3.8 cm

段枝状，表面有轻度风化。为古代香料之一，用东南亚所产檀香木枝干制成。这批香料来源于 1973 年 8 月在福建泉州湾后渚港发掘出土的一艘宋代海船中。

中华医学会／上海中医药大学医史博物馆藏

The spice is shaped like a tree branch and its surface is slightly weathered. As one type of the ancient spices in Southeast Asia, it is made of sandalwood branches. The spice came from a Song Dynasty ship which was excavated in Houzhu Port, Quanzhou Bay, Fujian Province, in August 1973.

Preserved in Chinese Medical Association/ Museum of Chinese Medicine, Shanghai University of Traditional Chinese Medicine

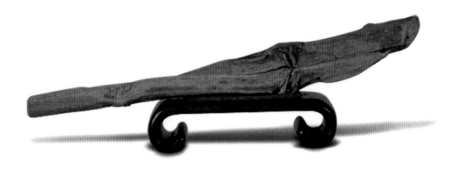

香料

宋

木质

长 25 厘米，宽 3 厘米

Spice

Song Dynasty

Wood

Length 25 cm/ Width 3 cm

段枝状，表面有轻度风化。为古代香料之一，用东南亚所产檀香木枝干制成。这批香料来源于 1973 年 8 月在福建泉州湾后渚港发掘出土的一艘宋代海船中。

中华医学会 / 上海中医药大学医史博物馆藏

The spice is shaped like a tree branch and its surface is slightly weathered. As one type of the ancient spices in Southeast Asia, it is made of sandalwood branches. The spice came from a Song Dynasty ship which was excavated in Houzhu Port, Quanzhou Bay, Fujian Province, in August 1973.

Preserved in Chinese Medical Association/ Museum of Chinese Medicine, Shanghai University of Traditional Chinese Medicine

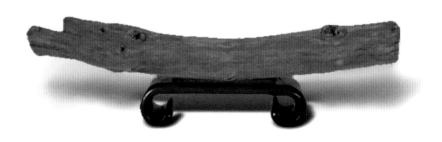

香料

宋

木质

长 26.2 厘米，宽 3.2 厘米

Spice

Song Dynasty

Wood

Length 26.2 cm/ Width 3.2 cm

段枝状，表面有轻度风化。为古代香料之一，用东南亚所产檀香木枝干制成。这批香料来源于 1973 年 8 月在福建泉州湾后渚港发掘出土的一艘宋代海船中。

中华医学会 / 上海中医药大学医史博物馆藏

The spice is shaped like a tree branch and its surface is slightly weathered. As one type of the ancient spices in Southeast Asia, it is made of sandalwood branches. The spice came from a Song Dynasty ship which was excavated in Houzhu Port, Quanzhou Bay, Fujian Province, in August 1973.

Preserved in Chinese Medical Association/ Museum of Chinese Medicine, Shanghai University of Traditional Chinese Medicine

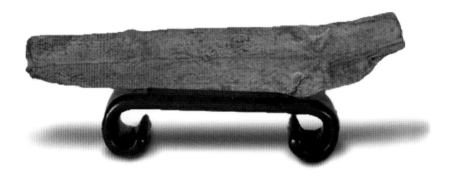

香料

宋

木质

长 18.5 厘米，宽 3.1 厘米

Spice

Song Dynasty

Wood

Length 18.5 cm/ Width 3.1 cm

段枝状，表面有轻度风化。为古代香料之一，
用东南亚所产檀香木枝干制成。这批香料来源
于 1973 年 8 月在福建泉州湾后渚港发掘出土
的一艘宋代海船中。

中华医学会 / 上海中医药大学医史博物馆藏

The spice is shaped like a tree branch and its
surface is slightly weathered. As one type of
the ancient spices in Southeast Asia, it is made
of sandalwood branches. The spice came from
a Song Dynasty ship which was excavated in
Houzhu Port, Quanzhou Bay, Fujian Province, in
August 1973.

Preserved in Chinese Medical Association/ Museum
of Chinese Medicine, Shanghai University of
Traditional Chinese Medicine

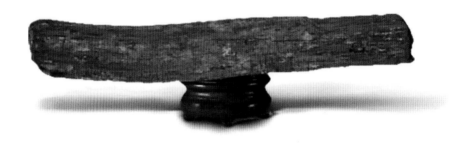

香料

宋

木质

长 13.9 厘米，宽 2 厘米

Spice

Song Dynasty

Wood

Length 13.9 cm/ Width 2 cm

段枝状，表面有轻度风化。为古代香料之一，用东南亚所产檀香木枝干制成。这批香料来源于 1973 年 8 月在福建泉州湾后渚港发掘出土的一艘宋代海船中。

中华医学会 / 上海中医药大学医史博物馆藏

The spice is shaped like a tree branch and its surface is slightly weathered. As one type of the ancient spices in Southeast Asia, it is made of sandalwood branches. The spice came from a Song Dynasty ship which was excavated in Houzhu Port, Quanzhou Bay, Fujian Province, in August 1973.

Preserved in Chinese Medical Association/ Museum of Chinese Medicine, Shanghai University of Traditional Chinese Medicine

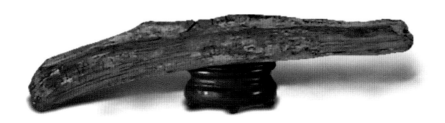

香料

宋

木质

长 13.9 厘米，宽 2 厘米

Spice

Song Dynasty

Wood

Length 13.9 cm/ Width 2 cm

段枝状，表面有轻度风化。为古代香料之一，用东南亚所产檀香木枝干制成。这批香料来源于 1973 年 8 月在福建泉州湾后渚港发掘出土的一艘宋代海船中。

中华医学会 / 上海中医药大学医史博物馆藏

The spice is shaped like a tree branch and its surface is slightly weathered. As one type of the ancient spices in Southeast Asia, it is made of sandalwood branches. The spice came from a Song Dynasty ship which was excavated in Houzhu Port, Quanzhou Bay, Fujian Province, in August 1973. Preserved in Chinese Medical Association/ Museum of Chinese Medicine, Shanghai University of Traditional Chinese Medicine

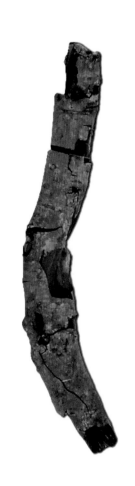

香料

宋

木质

长 32 厘米，宽 3.9 厘米

Spice

Song Dynasty

Wood

Length 32 cm/ Width 3.9 cm

段枝状，表面有轻度风化。为古代香料之一，用东南亚所产檀香木枝干制成。这批香料来源于 1973 年 8 月在福建泉州湾后渚港发掘出土的一艘宋代海船中。

中华医学会 / 上海中医药大学医史博物馆藏

The spice is shaped like a tree branch and its surface is slightly weathered. As one type of the ancient spices in Southeast Asia, it is made of sandalwood branches. The spice came from a Song Dynasty ship which was excavated in Houzhu Port, Quanzhou Bay, Fujian Province, in August 1973. Preserved in Chinese Medical Association/ Museum of Chinese Medicine, Shanghai University of Traditional Chinese Medicine

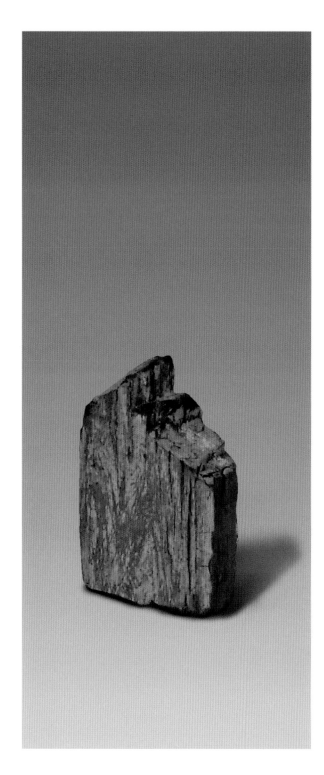

香料

宋

木质

长 6.6 厘米，宽 3.9 厘米

Spice

Song Dynasty

Wood

Length 6.6 cm/ Width 3.9 cm

段枝状，表面有轻度风化。为古代香料之一，
用东南亚所产檀香木枝干制成。这批香料来源
于 1973 年 8 月在福建泉州湾后渚港发掘出土
的一艘宋代海船中。

中华医学会 / 上海中医药大学医史博物馆藏

The spice is shaped like a tree branch and its surface
is slightly weathered. As one type of the ancient
spices in Southeast Asia, it is made of sandalwood
branches. The spice came from a Song Dynasty
ship which was excavated in Houzhu Port,
Quanzhou Bay, Fujian Province, in August 1973.
Preserved in Chinese Medical Association/ Museum
of Chinese Medicine, Shanghai University of
Traditional Chinese Medicine

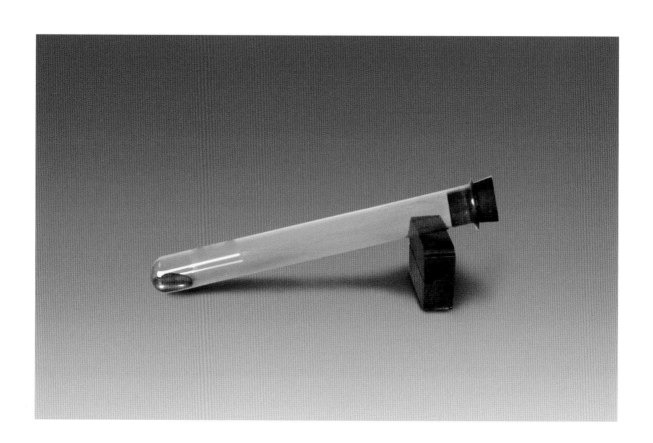

水银

宋

矿物

约 0.5 毫升

Mercury

Song Dynasty

Mineral

Volume about 0.5 mL

宋代残存至今的医用水银，呈液状。用试管保存，基本完好。福建省博物馆调拨，1978 年入藏。

中华医学会 / 上海中医药大学医史博物馆藏

The collection was liquid mercury for medical use conserved from the Song Dynasty. It was kept in a test tube in basically intact condition. It was collected by the Fujian Museum in 1978.

Preserved in Chinese Medical Association/ Museum of Chinese Medicine, Shanghai University of Traditional Chinese Medicine

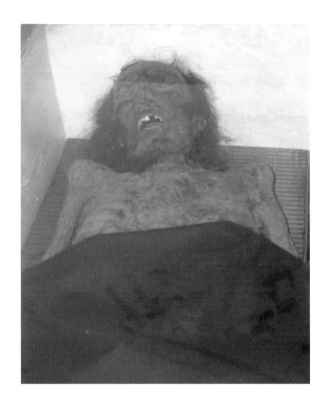

干尸

明

古尸

高 164 厘米

Mummy

Ming Dynasty

Ancient Corpse

Height 164 cm

为成年男性干燥尸体，体表皮肤完整，眉毛、头发、胡子、牙齿等均完好存在，稍有残。宁夏回族自治区中卫县（今中卫市）出土，1978 年入藏。

陕西医史博物馆藏

The mummy is an adult man's dry cadaver. The surface of the skin, hair, beard, eyebrows, and teeth are in good condition except for being slightly incomplete. The mummy was excavated in Zhongwei County (now Zhongwei City), Ningxia Hui Autonomous Region and was collected in the museum in 1978.

Preserved in Shaanxi Museum of Medical History

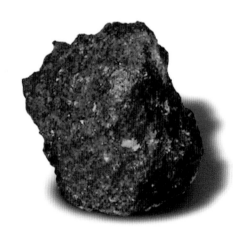

云母

明

矿物

长 4.6 厘米，宽 2.5 厘米，厚 5.2 厘米

Mica

Ming Dynasty

Mineral

Length 4.6 cm/ Width 2.5 cm/ Thickness 5.2 cm

块状云母矿，为明万历年（1573—1620）遗物，共计三块，表面有轻度风化。药用。苏州市博物馆捐赠，1976 年入藏。

中华医学会 / 上海中医药大学医史博物馆藏

The collection, which was made in Wanli Period (1573–1620) of the Ming Dynasty, is of massive structure and consists of three pieces in total. Its surface is slightly weathered. The mica was used as a drug. Suzhou Museum donated it. It was collected in the museum in 1976.
Preserved in Chinese Medical Association/ Museum of Chinese Medicine, Shanghai University of Traditional Chinese Medicine

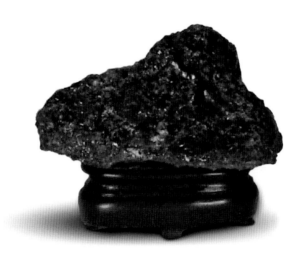

云母

明

矿物

长 5.3 厘米，宽 2.6 厘米，厚 2.6 厘米

Mica

Ming Dynasty

Mineral

Length 5.3 cm/ Width 2.6 cm/ Thickness 2.6 cm

块状云母矿，为明万历年遗物，共计三块，表面有轻度风化。药用。苏州市博物馆捐赠，1976年入藏。

中华医学会/上海中医药大学医史博物馆藏

The collection, which was made in Wanli Period of the Ming Dynasty, is of massive structure and has three pieces in total. Its surface is slightly weathered. It was used as a drug. Suzhou Museum donated it. It was collected in the museum in 1976.

Preserved in Chinese Medical Association/ Museum of Chinese Medicine, Shanghai University of Traditional Chinese Medicine

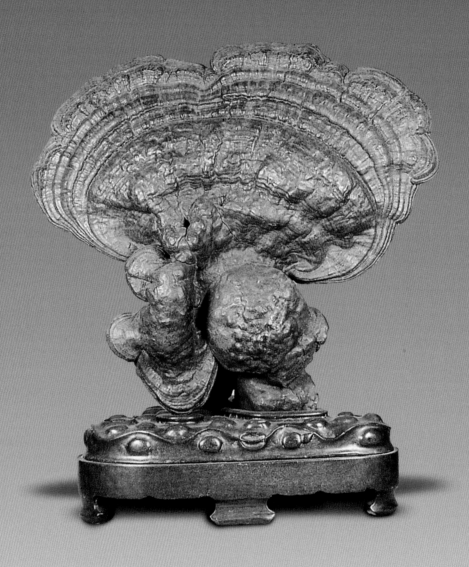

灵芝标本

清

植物

宽 43 厘米，高 20 厘米

为紫芝，黑褐色，有细孔，质坚硬光滑。

上海中医药博物馆藏

Ganoderma Specimen

Qing Dynasty

Plant

Width 43 cm/ Height 20 cm

The color of this ganoderma is black brown. There are some fine pores on the surface. The texture of the specimen is hard and smooth. Preserved in Shanghai Museum of Traditional Chinese Medicine

索 引

（馆藏地按拼音字母排序）

邹城市文物局

Index

Zoucheng Municipal Bureau of Cultural Relics

参考文献

[1] 李经纬.中国古代医史图录 [M].北京：人民卫生出版社，1992.

[2] 傅维康，李经纬，林昭庚.中国医学通史：文物图谱卷 [M].北京：人民卫生出版社，2000.

[3] 和中浚，吴鸿洲.中华医学文物图集 [M].成都：四川人民出版社，2001.

[4] 上海中医药博物馆.上海中医药博物馆馆藏珍品 [M].上海：上海科学技术出版社，2013.

[5] 西藏自治区博物馆.西藏博物馆 [M].北京：五洲传播出版社，2005.

[6] 崔乐泉.中国古代体育文物图录：中英文本 [M].北京：中华书局，2000.

[7] 张金明，陆雪春.中国古铜镜鉴赏图录 [M].北京：中国民族摄影艺术出版社，2002.

[8] 文物精华编辑委员会.文物精华 [M].北京：文物出版社，1964.

[9] 谭维四.湖北出土文物精华 [M].武汉：湖北教育出版社，2001.

[10] 常州市博物馆.常州文物精华 [M].北京：文物出版社，1998.

[11] 镇江博物馆.镇江文物精华 [M].合肥：黄山书社，1997.

[12] 贵州省文化厅，贵州省博物馆.贵州文物精华 [M].贵阳：贵州人民出版社，2005.

[13] 徐良玉.扬州馆藏文物精华 [M].南京：江苏古籍出版社，2001.

[14] 昭陵博物馆，陕西历史博物馆.昭陵文物精华 [M].西安：陕西人民美术出版社，1991.

[15] 南通博物苑.南通博物苑文物精华 [M].北京：文物出版社，2005.

[16] 邯郸市文物研究所.邯郸文物精华 [M].北京：文物出版社，2005.

[17] 张秀生，刘友恒，聂连顺，等.中国河北正定文物精华 [M].北京：文化艺术出版社，1998.

[18] 陕西省咸阳市文物局.咸阳文物精华 [M].北京：文物出版社，2002.

[19] 安阳市文物管理局.安阳文物精华 [M].北京：文物出版社，2004.

[20] 深圳市博物馆.深圳市博物馆文物精华 [M].北京：文物出版社，1998.

[21]《中国文物精华》编辑委员会.中国文物精华（1993）[M].北京：文物出版社，1993.

[22] 夏路，刘永生．山西省博物馆馆藏文物精华 [M]．太原：山西人民出版社，1999．

[23] 文物精华编辑委员会．文物精华 [M]．北京：文物出版社，1957．

[24] 山西博物院，湖北省博物馆．荆楚长歌：九连墩楚墓出土文物精华 [M]．太原：山西人民出版社，2011．

[25] 刘广堂，石金鸣，宋建忠．晋国雄风：山西出土两周文物精华 [M]．沈阳：万卷出版公司，2009．

[26] 沈君山，王国平，单迎红．滦平博物馆馆藏文物精华 [M]．北京：中国文联出版社，2012．

[27] 张家口市博物馆．张家口市博物馆馆藏文物精华 [M]．北京：科学出版社，2011．

[28] 浙江省文物考古研究所．浙江考古精华 [M]．北京：文物出版社，1999．

[29] 故宫博物院．故宫雕刻珍萃 [M]．北京：紫禁城出版社，2004．

[30] 故宫博物院紫禁城出版社．故宫博物院藏宝录 [M]．上海：上海文艺出版社，1986．

[31] 首都博物馆．大元三都 [M]．北京：科学出版社，2016．

[32] 新疆维吾尔自治区博物馆．新疆出土文物 [M]．北京：文物出版社，1975．

[33] 王兴伊，段逸山．新疆出土涉医文书辑校 [M]．上海：上海科学技术出版社，2016．

[34] 刘学春．刍议医药卫生文物的概念与分类标准 [J]．中华中医药杂志，2016，31（11）:4406–4409．

[35] 上海古籍出版社．中国艺海 [M]．上海：上海古籍出版社，1994．

[36] 紫都，岳鑫．一生必知的 200 件国宝 [M]．呼和浩特：远方出版社，2005．

[37] 谭维四．湖北出土文物精华 [M]．武汉：湖北教育出版社，2001．

[38] 张建青．青海彩陶收藏与鉴赏 [M]．北京：中国文史出版社，2007．

[39] 银景琦．仡佬族文物 [M]．南宁：广西人民出版社，2014．

[40] 廖果，梁峻，李经纬．东西方医学的反思与前瞻 [M]．北京：中医古籍出版社，2002．

[41] 梁峻，张志斌，廖果，等．中华医药文明史集论 [M]．北京：中医古籍出版社，2003．

[42] 郑蓉，庄乾竹，刘聪，等．中国医药文化遗产考论 [M]．北京：中医古籍出版社，2005．